... born in Kirkby, Merseyside, ... 1971 and made his league debut for Bolton Wanderers as a teenager. Having helped the club through two promotions to the Premier League, he was subsequently signed by Celtic in 1996 for a fee of over £4 million. After beating two bouts of cancer, Stubbs moved south in 2001 to join the team he had supported as a boy, Everton. He eventually retired in 2008, having made almost 500 league appearances in his career, before joining the club's coaching staff. He still lives on Merseyside with his wife Mandy and their two children, Heather and Sam.

**Tom Bromley**, who worked with Alan Stubbs on the writing of this book, was born in Salisbury in 1972, and grew up in York. A publisher and writer, he is the ghost of six previous books, including *Sunday Times* top ten bestsellers, and the author of eight further titles in his own right. He now lives in Salisbury with his wife and their two children.

# HOW FOOTBALL SAVED MY LIFE

ALAN STUBBS

with Tom Bromley

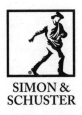

**SIMON &
SCHUSTER**

London · New York · Sydney · Toronto · New Delhi

A CBS COMPANY

First published in Great Britain by Simon & Schuster UK Ltd, 2013
This paperback edition published by Simon & Schuster UK Ltd, 2014

A CBS company

1 3 5 7 9 10 8 6 4 2

Simon & Schuster UK Ltd
1st Floor
222 Gray's Inn Road
London WC1X 8HB

www.simonandschuster.co.uk

Simon & Schuster Australia,
Sydney

Simon & Schuster India,
New Delhi

A CIP catalogue record for this book is available from the British Library

ISBN: 978-1-47112-834-9
Ebook ISBN: 978-47112-835-6

Typeset in the UK by Hewer Text UK Ltd, Edinburgh
Printed and bound by CPI Group (UK) Ltd, Croydon, CR0 4YY

*To Mandy, for being such a brilliant wife
and mum and for putting up with me.*

# Contents

# 1

‘Listen, Alan. I’ve got
some bad news for you.’

The last thing I wanted to do after losing a cup final was to be frogmarched off to do a drugs test.

The 1999 Scottish Cup final had been my first taste of that special Hampden atmosphere, but for all the excitement and build-up preceding the match, it was rapidly leaving a bittersweet taste in my mouth. So many of my friends and family had come up from Liverpool to soak up the occasion, but all they had witnessed was the despair of an agonising Celtic defeat. Now, rather than being allowed to share my disappointment with my team-mates, my only post-match companions were to be a doping agent and a small glass jar.

It had not been a good season to be a Celtic player. Rangers had already won the League Cup, and then the championship title in a toxic Old Firm match at Parkhead. That match had threatened to spiral out of control both on and off the pitch: three players had been dismissed and another ten yellow carded as tempers frayed; the referee Hugh Dallas had to have medical treatment after being struck by a coin from a fan. ‘Ninety Minutes of Pure Poison' was one of the newspaper headlines the next day, and for once the press weren't exaggerating. Dallas, who'd done his best to keep a lid on the game, had been chosen again as referee for the cup final. I hoped that was not going to be an omen of how things were going to go.

The white-hot intensity of an Old Firm match is difficult to describe if you've never been part of one. I played in twenty-four such games over my time at Celtic, and let me tell you, they're not for the faint-hearted. Occasionally, a game of football emerged, and the many talents of both sides managed to shine through. But more often than not the sun went in, and they degenerated into something closer to a kicking competition – one in which the ref had to turn a blind eye in order to keep enough players on the pitch. All of this frenzied football was conducted in a cacophony of noise and passion like I've never heard – the venom of the terrace chants threatening to spill over onto the pitch at any moment. I'd been playing that day in 1998 when Gazza had done his 'flute playing' in front of the Celtic fans. That had been tinder-box stuff, and the fall out from that was not something anyone wanted to see repeated.

An Old Firm cup final was unique because it was the only time that Celtic and Rangers fans were at a match in equal numbers. At Parkhead and Ibrox, the terraces were stacked one way or the other: Hampden was fifty-fifty between our supporters and theirs. That made for a cracking atmosphere, if for a policing headache. There was none of the usual intermingling of fans on the way to the stadium you get down Wembley Way: none of that fan-friendly walking to the stadium together in the warm spring sunshine. Instead, the green and white hoops of Celtic and the blue of Rangers were kept well away from each other by lines of mounted police. The two sets of supporters were shepherded to the stadium from opposite directions: the first sight they caught of their rival fans was in the ground itself, where they made up for lost time by doubling up their shouting and chanting.

I was one of those footballers for whom winning is the be all and end all. Once I'm on the pitch, that's it. That's all I want to do. I would throw myself into every challenge, stretch every last sinew to achieve that. I've never been one of those who could comfort themselves by thinking, 'we lost but we played the better football'. All I would think was 'we lost'. That day, I was desperate to win the match several times over: because it was a cup final, because it was Rangers, because they were on course for a treble, because I hated to lose. On top of that, I was acutely aware it was the last match of the season. Get beat, and I'd be leaving for my summer holidays with that sour taste of losing in my mouth. There'd be no chance to make amends, and plenty of opportunity to fester on the beach about what could and should have been.

The 1999 Cup final wasn't the frenzied atmosphere of the Old Firm match we'd played a few weeks earlier. Instead, it was one of those taut, tight, tense affairs, where there wasn't so much as a cigarette paper between the two sides. Both teams were determined to dig in and defend like their lives depended on it – manning the barricades and squeezing the breath out of the opposition. It wasn't until the second half that the deadlock was broken. Rangers' Tony Vidmar had crossed the ball into the Celtic penalty area from the left, to where Neil McCann was waiting. I was right there, had read exactly what was going to happen, and threw myself in to block the shot. Rather than the ball rocketing goalwards, it ricocheted off my leg and squirrelled away into the path of Rod Wallace. It could have dropped anywhere, but the luck wasn't with me, and it fell perfectly for him. Wallace didn't turn that sort of opportunity down, and tucked the ball beyond our keeper, cool as you like. I groaned. One-nil Rangers, and the blue half of the stadium went ballistic.

The heads didn't go down: if anything, going a goal behind only spurred us on further, and we gave it everything to get back on level terms. I found myself piling forwards from defence: it was like a throwback to my schoolboy days, when my original position had been higher up the pitch. I was giving it everything I had, mixing it up in their penalty area in the hope of getting a nick or a chance, then sprinting back to defend our goal as Rangers mounted another assault. Sixty-five minutes in, I got my opportunity to equalise as the ball fell to me on the edge of the penalty area. I fired off one shot, which Colin Hendry took the full force of, collapsing to the floor in a heap. The ball bounced back off his body towards me and I shot again. This time, it took a great save from the Rangers keeper to keep the ball out. On eighty-seven minutes, in the face of more relentless Celtic pressure, Lorenzo Amoruso blocked another goal-bound shot with what looked suspiciously like his arm. The green and white half of Hampden went crazy: to us, it was a definite penalty. Here we go, I thought: it's the equaliser and extra-time now. But the referee Hugh Dallas was completely unmoved and waved our protests away. Maybe he'd had his fill of Old Firm derbies for the season, and wasn't going to extend the occasion any longer than he had to. A couple of minutes later, he blew up for full-time.

I felt gutted, shattered, drained. Cup finals are often the matches when players go down with cramp, and playing in one, it's easy to see why. There's the extra heat of the end of season sunshine, the additional pressure of the occasion, and the ferocious intensity of the football. You're giving absolutely everything you've got: for the team, for the fans. If you're not close to dropping at the end of all that, you shouldn't have been on the pitch in the first place. Of course, if you win, none of that matters: lifting the trophy has this miraculous effect of making you forget about your aches and pain. If you don't, however, there's nothing to distract you from how bad your body is feeling.

I never liked to lose, especially against Rangers, and especially when I felt we'd deserved something out of the match. It was a wrench to watch their victory celebrations. When Rangers had beaten Celtic to win the title at Parkhead, the players had celebrated their victory by doing a mock version of our team huddle, which was a longstanding part of the Celtic match routine. This time, it was their fans who infuriated me. As we went up to get our losers' medals – they're not runners-up medals, whatever anyone says – the Rangers supporters were heckling and goading us. I'd had enough. I responded with what one paper euphemistically described as a 'one-handed salute': I gave them the well-known 'Gareth Hunt' hand gesture from the Nescafé TV commercial – and I wasn't suggesting they went off and made a cup of coffee! Unfortunately, my actions were picked up by the TV cameras and the story was all over the papers the next day. It was not a great moment all round.

I just wanted to get out of there, to be honest. But my bad day at the office was about to get worse. As I came back down the steps, there was a guy in a suit standing waiting for me. He was from the UK Doping Agency, and along with my team-mate Enrico Annoni, I'd been chosen to take a drugs test. You never know when these agents are going to turn up: it was random which matches they'd be at, and whether it was your turn. The odds of being picked, therefore, were quite small – it's got a bit tighter now, but back then I reckon I'd get tested once or twice a season at most. When the agent told me it was my turn, it wouldn't surprise me if I'd given him a look. Not because I didn't believe in testing, but because it meant that rather than going back into the dressing room with my team-mates, to digest the match and talk about it together, I was to be escorted off to give a urine sample.

I knew from experience that producing that was no quick call. This might sound a stupid thing, but it's difficult to have a piss after a match because you're so dehydrated. As a defender, you'd normally be covering between nine and a half and ten and a half kilometres a match, losing several litres of fluid in the process. You lose so much during a game that you're encouraged to take on as much fluid as possible in the day or so before to compensate. So it might sound a simple thing to do, to give a urine sample, but it can take an absolute age. Sometimes they even try giving you a beer or two to speed things up.

I was sat there mulling over the match, still in my kit and boots, desperate to talk to the lads, and unable to go. It wasn't the way I wanted to finish the day or the season, but that's how it was. I'm not the sort to naturally feel sorry for myself, but there was nothing to do but sit there and stew. In the end it was about an hour and a half before I could pass water. I did my two samples – you have to do a couple in case one of them is negative. The drugs testers aren't allowed to touch them in case of contamination, so you screw the jars shut yourself, put them in a polystyrene satchel, seal it and sign to say it's all your own work.

I was lucky: the team bus, which had been about to depart, was still there when I was done. Another few minutes, and they'd have gone without me. That happened to Enrico who still hadn't produced a sample at this point: he'd have to make his own way home. I piled on the bus with my team-mates, pleased to see the back of Hampden. I was looking forward to forgetting about the afternoon, and starting to think about some recuperation and my summer break. The coach pulled away from the stadium, and that was the last I thought about the drugs test.

Three weeks later, I was back down in Liverpool. The disappointments of the end of the season were now a distant memory: I'd been abroad with Mandy and the kids (Heather, who was three, and Sam, who was seven months old at the time), and had enjoyed what felt like a well-deserved bit of sunshine. Mandy and I were both from Merseyside, so the close season was always a good time to head back down the M6 and catch up with family and friends. That particular Tuesday it was warm and sunny, and I was out on the golf course, playing a few holes with Mark Seagraves, my former Bolton Wanderers team-mate, and a friend of his. I enjoy my golf – I play off seven – and life felt good. The putts were rolling in, the sun was out and the company was great. I was thinking ahead to the new season, and chatting with Mark about working with the new Celtic managerial team of Director of Football Kenny Dalglish and coach John Barnes. Funny how I'd almost signed for Dalglish at Blackburn, and now here he was – my boss after all.

We were well into the back nine when my phone rang. We must have been on the twelfth or fourteenth, something like that – I can't remember exactly, but it would have been appropriate if it had been the thirteenth hole, given what the call was about. In those days I had one of those flip-top phones that you open up, and was surprised to find Jack Mulhearn, the Celtic doctor, on the other end of the line.

'Hi Alan,' he said, 'How are things?'

'Yeah, good,' I replied.

'How are you feeling?' he asked.

Strange question, I remember thinking. 'Yeah,' I said. 'I feel great.'

'Okay,' Jack said. 'That's good.'

Then he paused. It was quite a long pause, an unsettling one, like he was trying to work out the best way to phrase things.

'Listen Alan,' Jack continued. 'I've got some bad news for you. It's the drugs test you did. After the cup final.'

7

'You what?' This conversation was getting stranger by the second.

'It's come back positive Alan.'

For a second or two, I was speechless. Had I heard him right? I was completely dumbfounded.

'That's impossible,' I said eventually. And it was. I'd never taken anything in my life. I'd had my opportunities – as did any modern footballer on a night out – but it was something that had never remotely interested me.

'I know,' said Jack. He sounded a little relieved by my answer. 'I'm sorry I have to ask you these questions, but you know how it is. So you're saying you haven't been taking anything?'

'Come on,' I said. 'You know me Jack. You know I wouldn't do anything like that.'

'I know that,' said Jack, 'and I'm sorry. But I had to ask.' He paused again. 'Okay. The thing is, Alan, there's no doubt you've failed the test. What it's showing is that you're producing a high level of a hormone that is usually only found in pregnant woman . . .'

At this point, I was still thinking that there must have been a bizarre mix up somewhere along the line. Pregnant women? It still didn't make any sense.

'. . . when it's found in men, it's for a different reason,' Jack continued. 'The only time this hormone is found in a man, and there's no easy way of saying this, is when it's linked to testicular cancer.'

That was a jolt, I can tell you. I hadn't seen that coming at all. Cancer.

'OK,' I said, a little dazed. I breathed out. 'Bloody hell.'

'Have you, er . . . checked yourself lately?' Jack asked. His voice was more serious now. 'Have you come across any lumps or anything like that?'

As soon he said that, I just knew. 'Now that you mention it, I have had a bit of pain in one my testicles, my left one.'

'How long have you had that for?'

'Not long,' I said. 'Couple of months, maybe. It's just something that has come and gone, you know. I didn't really think anything about it.'

'Well, we need to get it checked, Alan,' Jack said. 'As a priority.'

Like any footballer, I was used to getting aches and pains the whole time. Cuts and bruises, they came with the territory. I'd always been the sort of player to throw myself into challenges, whatever the consequences: I'd had broken collarbones and fractured cheekbones over the years for my troubles, so by contrast the dull ache in my balls was something I hadn't really taken much notice of. I remembered having a feel when I first noticed, and thinking that one of my testicles seemed different to the other. There wasn't a noticeable lump or anything like that: it was just a bit hard. I've got to be honest and say that I'd thought no more about it. At the time I didn't really know anything about testicular cancer, or what the symptoms were.

Certainly, I hadn't felt ill or anything like that. Far from it: I was twenty-eight and at the top of my game. I ate a healthy diet and went to the gym every day: at the club, I was known for being one of the fitter ones. As a professional footballer, you had your performance level checked the whole time, so even if I'd been a bit off colour, I would have known about it straightaway. But nothing like that had come up: as far as I was concerned, I was in the best shape of my life.

'Who was that?' Mark asked, after I'd hung up the phone.

'The club doctor,' I said. 'He thinks I might have testicular cancer.'

'You what?' Mark looked at me as though I was joking.

'I know.' But I didn't know. Not really. Not yet.

'Come on,' Mark said, realising I was serious. He started putting his club back in his bag. 'We'll go.'

'No,' I replied. 'There's nothing I can do about it now. Let's finish the round.'

I was insistent on that. Maybe it was a coping mechanism, to carry on as normal. We played the remaining holes, not that I could tell you much about them. The decent round I'd started on the outward nine quickly degenerated as my mind began to wander. Then I went home, to try and tell my wife and my family what the doctor had said.

On Thursday morning, Mandy and I were driven up to Glasgow, in a car provided by the club. A few years earlier, in 1996, I'd made the same journey in somewhat different circumstances. Celtic had made an offer of £4.5 million to make me their record signing, and I was going up to meet the then manager, Tommy Burns, and discuss personal terms. I'd been a Bolton Wanderers player for several years by this point, and was more than ready for the move. I'd almost signed for Kenny Dalglish's Premier League winning Blackburn the year before, in a £9 million double deal with my Bolton team-mate Jason McAteer. But then Liverpool had come in for Jason, his childhood club, and the deal was pulled.

The Celtic offer was an amazing opportunity, but it wasn't the only one on the table. My former manager at Bolton, Bruce Rioch, was now in charge at Arsenal, and he was desperate for me to come and play for him at Highbury. When he got wind of the Celtic deal, he was absolutely insistent: don't sign anything until I've spoken to you, he said. The fee, the personal terms, none of that will be a problem. Just don't agree the contract until you've had my call.

That day, driving up to Glasgow with my agent, we couldn't have gone any slower. We drove at fifty miles an hour up the M6 in the slow lane with the lorries, stopping off at one service station after another for a coffee, then again at the next one for a toilet break. I was completely torn about what I wanted: Arsenal and Celtic were both enormous clubs, but I couldn't ignore the possibility of working with Bruce again. He was the manager who'd always believed in me, and had helped make me the player I was. If there was a chance of renewing that relationship, I couldn't just dismiss it out of hand, however much the prospect of playing for Celtic excited me.

Finally, about fifteen miles south of Glasgow, Bruce rang. The news wasn't good.

'Listen,' he said. 'I've got some problems here. You should go and sign for Celtic. I'm really disappointed, but it's not going to happen here, I'm afraid.'

Later, it transpired that Rioch had been having problems with his striker Ian Wright, a fractious relationship that was to threaten his position. It wasn't long afterwards that he was sacked and replaced by Arsene Wenger. By then, however, I'd been more than blown away by Celtic. As soon as I'd got there that day, I'd been warmly welcomed by Tommy Burns, who took me round and showed me the stadium. I came out of the tunnel onto the pitch, and just thought, wow. I tried to imagine what it would be like, playing in front of 62,000 passionate fans, and knew there and then that this was the club for me. I fell in love with the ground, with the history and with the friendliness I encountered: it was like the family club atmosphere I'd been used to at Bolton, but everything was ten times the size.

That was then, though, and this was now. Waiting for Bruce Rioch's call, I'd wanted the journey up the M6 to go on forever. This time round, however much the driver put his foot down in the fast lane, I couldn't get to Glasgow fast enough. Back then, the journey had all been about possibilities – multi-million pound transfers and where to spend the peak years of my footballing career. Now it was about how my life might unfold, but in a different way – the earlier sense of excitement replaced by something starker, more sombre.

This time round, there was no welcoming party on the front steps for me. I was driven round the side of Celtic Park and slipped in through the back door. The smiles of the staff were still there, but they were of the concerned, worried kind. I sat down with Jack, and we had a brief chat about my situation. He showed me a pile of books he'd been reading on the subject, and did everything he could to reassure me, and to downplay my concerns.

'I'm sure it's nothing,' he said. 'These are all just routine tests you're going to do.'

Mandy was asking him all sorts of questions, but Jack just said, 'Let's just hold those, until we know exactly what this is. There's no point worrying about something if it's not actually that.'

We drove from the ground to the Bon Secours Private Hospital, where Celtic did all their medical tests. I knew it well from the number of knee scans and the like I'd had over the years. Jack guided me through, and introduced me to the guy who was going to do my scan. Again, he couldn't have been friendlier. He led me into a room, where I took my clothes off, and put on a gown. Then I sat on a bed and waited for the ultrasound.

The procedure and machine were exactly the same as when a pregnant woman has a scan: for a moment, it brought back memories of when I'd been to the hospital with Mandy, when she was pregnant with Heather and Sam. But the cold squeeze of the gel being smeared over my testicles brought me quickly back to reality. The doctor ran the machine over my right testicle first, and we both looked over at the screen, to see what it was showing up. The image of my testicle was all grey, like a light white-grey egg.

'That's all good,' the doctor said. 'Looks clear to me. There's no problem with that at all.'

Then he moved the scanner round to my other testicle. Immediately you could see the difference. This time, the 'egg' was three-quarters black. I remember thinking it looked a little like a new moon, with a light grey crescent on one side, and the darkness spreading out from the opposite side.

'That's it,' the doctor said, simply. 'That's the problem, right there.'

I felt shocked, of course I did. But at the same time, in a curious way that shock was mixed with relief. If I was being honest with myself, there had been something in the back of my mind, even before the drugs test, that something wasn't quite right. I'd tried to ignore it, but that sense of unease had never quite gone away. Then, since the phone call with Jack on the golf course, I'd been left with that horrible sense of uncertainty. I wasn't someone who liked that: if I knew what the score was, however bad the situation, then I could face up and deal with it. It was the not knowing that really gnawed away at me.

The day was turning into something of a whirlwind. From Merseyside to Glasgow, from Celtic Park to the hospital, and now straight from the ultrasound straight in to see the specialist. He took a look at the scans, and spoke with the same certainty as the doctor who had done the scan.

'It's testicular cancer,' he said, after looking carefully at the pictures. 'What we don't know at this stage is what type.'

I'd known next to nothing about testicular cancer before the drugs test, but now I found myself catching up fast. There were two types of testicular cancer, essentially: there was a teratoma, which was an active and aggressive form of cancer, and likely to spread to other parts of the body; then there was a seminoma, which sat there dormant, like a volcano. It could trigger at any moment, but caught early, it could be removed before it had chance to spread.

'So which one have I got?' I asked.

'I'd love to be able to tell you,' the specialist said, 'but we won't know until after we've removed it. We'll then do a biopsy and should have the results back within a week. As for the operation,' he continued, 'it's a bit like a hernia. We'll cut just below the belly area, and force the testicle through the tubes, and bring it out that way. Is there anything you'd like to ask?'

My question was instinctive: 'When will I be able to play football again?'

That was my reaction. The specialist looked a little taken aback. This obviously wasn't the usual response he got when he told people they had cancer. But that was my mindset. I was a professional footballer: I felt invincible. The will to win that infused my game would see me through here as well: testicular cancer was just another opponent for me to face and which would get the same short shrift as a Rangers striker bearing down on goal.

The specialist smiled. 'It shouldn't be too long. You're probably looking at four to six weeks.'

I was surprised at how short the recovery time was, but immediately my thoughts whirred through more practical matters. Four to six weeks? I went through the dates. It was the end of June, so if I had the operation immediately, I might be back up and playing by the start of the next season.

'Let's get it done,' I said. The quicker I could have the operation, the quicker I would know exactly what it was I was dealing with.

In my head, I was completely focused on Celtic, and on my football. That was a sportsman's mentality, and it was a huge help in dealing with the situation. I was used to running out onto the pitch, and playing with the expectations of 62,000 people on my shoulders. That was pressure, and you needed to be strong psychologically not to crumple under that. I had that well of self-belief to draw from, and draw from it I did. It meant that when I first heard from Jack, and when the specialist confirmed I had testicular cancer, I didn't feel scared. I felt nervous and I felt helpless because I wasn't in control, but I didn't feel scared. The thought of death didn't once enter my mind at the time. It was only later that I came to understand just what a deadly opponent I was up against.

In the days before the operation, I got my first taste of how public a disease cancer can be. Just as the ultrasound scan had been a dark echo of the joy of pregnancy, so that weekend became the same sort of open house you have after the arrival of a newborn baby. Friends and family came down to see us from all corners of the country. Even though they all meant well, it was exhausting. I was still feeling okay and holding up, but the more people wished you luck and asked how you were, the stronger you had to be not to fall into feeling unwell, and lapsing into self-pity.

Just like on the football pitch, I found myself being the strong one. It was me who was carrying and supporting my relatives, not the other way round. It was my parents who I found most difficult discussing the situation with: I'd told my dad over the phone initially, because I knew if I'd done so face to face, I might not have been able to keep it together. Mandy's mum, meanwhile, had given me a hug and said, 'Oh, you'll be all right, Alan. You're a big strong lad.' Which we both knew was her way of saying 'Oh, shit'.

On the Monday before the operation, the press got wind of the story. Celtic had been brilliant in keeping things under wraps, but inevitably with something this big, it was going to leak out sooner or later. 'CELTIC STAR IN CANCER SCARE' ran the headline in the *Daily Record*: 'Cup Final Drugs Test Shows Up Need For Vital Op'. The story didn't name me in person, but said the player in question had been in the Celtic starting XI, and listed the team like a guessing game for the media. It didn't take long for journalists to work out it was me and start ringing up. That was the last thing I needed, so I got my agent to put out a statement, and asked for privacy.

The calls starting coming in, first from my Celtic team-mates, and then from players all round football. These conversations were good to have: they were concerned for me, but curious at the same time. How did I find it, what did it feel like, and so on. That was my first taste of how my illness might help others, and the public awareness of testicular cancer and its symptoms that might be raised by my own private battles.

By the Tuesday morning, when I was heading to the hospital for the operation, the story was all over the press, both north and south of the border. The newspapers were full of messages of support from both sides of the Old Firm divide: Rangers players like Scott Wilson and Sergio Porrini, former Ibrox favourites like Ally McCoist, as well as Celtic team-mates like Tommy Boyd and Henrik Larsson. The *Sun* even ran an editorial wishing me well: 'Stubbs is known for his unflagging determination and will to win as a player,' ran the 'Sun Says' piece. 'If he shows the same courage off the field as he does on it, there will only be one winner.'

I had a choice, meanwhile, as to whether or not to have a false testicle put in to replace the one that was about to be removed. The doctors had shown the sample to Mandy and me: it was like a small hard-boiled egg. It wouldn't have felt the same as a real testicle, but would have balanced things out in the mirror. It seemed quite a surreal conversation to be having, and when they'd shown it to us, we'd both burst out laughing. So I confirmed to the doctor that I'd rather just keep things the natural way. Out of everything that happened, that was probably the easiest decision I had to make.

I checked into the hospital in the morning as arranged. I was put under general anaesthetic and was in the operating theatre for just under an hour or so. The procedure went smoothly, so much so that rather than staying in overnight, I was allowed out at the end of the day. I was driven back to our house in Glasgow with strict instructions to relax and recuperate. I was a bit woozy from the anaesthetic and very uncomfortable for the first day or two: it was pretty sore down there, and I could feel it every time I stretched or sat up. But really, it felt no worse than recovering from any of the knocks I'd had on the pitch over the years.

What was really agony was the wait for the results of the biopsy. I'm not someone who is much good at sitting about doing nothing at the best of times. But to be in that position, to be under doctor's orders to put my feet up while waiting to find out what type of cancer it was, that was torture. I did my best to keep an open mind. I didn't want to think it was going to be a teratoma when it could be a seminoma. I'm a glass half-full, rather than a half-empty guy in life, and for those five days I did my best to stay an optimist.

By complete coincidence, on the Saturday after my operation, the 1999 Tour de France began with a prologue stage at Le Puy du Fou. I wasn't a huge cycling fan, but it was difficult not to notice who the winner was that day: a young American rider called Lance Armstrong, who was competing in the race for the first time since recovering from testicular cancer. Armstrong would go on to win that race, as well as the next six tours. His initial victory that day, as I was waiting for the biopsy results, only served to fuel my belief that I was going to pull through.

When the results came through, it was Jack who rang me.

'The biopsy has come back,' he told me down the phone. 'It's good news, Alan. It was a seminoma.'

Jack talked me through the report. When I'd first been diagnosed, they'd run tests to check the number of cancerous cells in the blood; a normal, healthy person would have a score of less than five: my reading had been seventy-eight. After the operation, this had fallen to twenty-five, and the expectation was that this would quickly fall back further. Not only that, but the cancer was still dormant when they'd taken it out. It was just sitting there, waiting to flare up. It could have triggered any day, but they'd removed it before it had chance.

I'd been very, very lucky. If the cup final hadn't been chosen by the doping agency as the game to run drugs tests, if I hadn't been picked at random as a player to be tested, the cancer would never have been detected.

I'd have gone off on my summer break completely ignorant of the situation: it could have been months before I'd been tested again, and who knows what might have happened by that point. I'd been extremely fortunate, or maybe it was something more than that: I'd devoted my entire life to football, and now, in return, football had saved my life.

I was elated. Absolutely overjoyed. It was the same shot of adrenaline sensation I'd had when I signed my first professional contract all those years before. I started the process of telling everyone the good news, thinking about pre-season and when I might get out on the pitch to hear the roar of the Celtic fans again. Little did I know then, but my battle with illness was only just beginning. Looking back now, my belief that those five days of waiting had been the worst of my life seems wishful thinking, to say the least. The cancer hadn't finished with me yet. In fact, it hadn't even begun. A footballer's mentality? Invincibility? Next time round, the cancer would strip me of all of that self-belief, and show me what it was really capable of. Next time round, I'd be fighting to stay alive.

# 2

## Striking for Pingwood

The biggest influence on my career was my dad, by far. Dad was the driving force behind my success. He was a football person, without actually being directly involved in football himself: he was a fan, an Evertonian, and knew the game inside out. He was the one who was on side and by my side everywhere I went. If it meant getting up at six o'clock in the morning to get to a match, then Dad was up at half five, getting me up to go. If it meant him getting off work early to take me to a game, then that's what he'd do. When I didn't really want to, Dad would never force me but just encourage in his own way.

'Come on son, we are going,' he'd say, quietly but firmly.

Without his support, I would never have achieved what I have.

It's only when you have children of your own that you understand just how much your parents did for you. I realise just how much I took all this for granted, and appreciate all the more what Dad did for me. Especially as there were so many of us for him and Mum to look after: I'm the youngest of five, my sister Susan is the eldest, then it's my brother Ronnie, Pam, Mandy and then me. I was the baby of the family, and the spoilt brat, so the others would say! I don't think I was: it just seemed that way as they were getting older. When they were the youngest one, I bet they got the attention, too.

Ronnie was a very good footballer when he was growing up. It's not easy for me to admit this, but technically, he was the better player. Ronnie played as a winger and had opportunities to go to clubs, if he'd wanted. He could have done well, but decided not to pursue them. Early on, he met his future wife, a Jehovah's Witness, and he decided that he wanted to go along that path rather than pursue a career in football. Growing up, I couldn't get my head round anyone not wanting to be a footballer if they had the chance. Now I'm older, I understand and totally respect him for what he did.

At the time, my dad was really disappointed by Ronnie's decision and was pretty cut up by it. He ended up not speaking to Ronnie, which looking back was a real shame. My mum was always the one who used to say, 'Let be'. For her, what Ronnie had done was not the end of the world and she would have quite happily got on with it. But my dad couldn't do that: he couldn't get beyond the fact that my brother had disappointed him. My mum was always loyal to my dad and so they didn't talk to Ronnie for quite a number of years. When they did speak again, it would still be frosty. If I could change anything, it would have been for my dad to forgive Ronnie sooner, before it was too late.

My parents were from Liverpool and from very working class backgrounds. We grew up in Kirkby, which was a tough place. If you didn't know the area and were to drive through it, you would look at Kirkby and dismiss it as somewhere not to hang about. For me, because I grew up there, I never really noticed any of that. It was home, and so it was normal. It was very much a working class area, with a lot of council housing. Yes, you had to know how to look after yourself, but it was also the sort of place where people would do everything for their family. They'd give their last penny to their children, and if it meant working three jobs to see them right, then that is what they'd do.

I love Kirkby and always will. If anyone has to say anything bad about it, I will always be the first one to stand up for it and fight its cause. I know the town has got its problems but I also know it has made me what I am today. I'm full of pride for where I have come from. Much of my family are still there too: my mum lives there, as do two of my sisters, with my brother and other sister just outside. We are all still in close proximity.

Kirkby is not a rich area. There are plenty of people on social care and benefits, and a lot of young people with children from an early age. You get those who make snide comments about who is paying for all this: Kirkby and Liverpool have had their knocks and the area has got its share of things that are not right. For some, Liverpool has got a stigma about it, all the rest of the country sees is people who rob and get involved in drugs, guns and gangs. I have got to say, though, that if I was to be anywhere and I was in trouble, I would want Liverpool people with me. I know if I was lost in Liverpool, someone would give me money to get home because it is the way they are.

They are a caring community and, for all the hardship, a generous community too. That is something that has always been the way, even from when I was a child through to today. My mum had two jobs and Dad had his job and if it meant them having five jobs to give us the best possible chance they could, then they would have done that. That was typical of Kirkby, of Liverpool and of Merseyside. It's that sort of spirit that makes it the amazing place it is.

\* \* \*

The house I grew up in was a three-bedroom semi, and felt a perfectly comfortable family home. Ronnie and I shared one room and slept in bunk beds: he was on the top and I was on the bottom. My sisters shared another room with three beds, and my parents had the other. So it suited us just fine. My dad worked for BAT, British American Tobacco. He was a driver's assistant and would travel round the country delivering cigarettes, doing the loading and unloading. He never drove the lorries himself: in fact, like my mum, he couldn't drive. It may have been because he couldn't afford a car, but as a result we were very much reliant on public transport. We'd go everywhere by bus and train, or get on our bikes to travel around.

Our street was a typical Merseyside one, with kids playing outside, kicking a football about and dreaming of playing for Everton or Liverpool. We'd use our gate as one goal, and someone else's as the other, and have a game. At least until someone came out and shouted: 'Get away! Go on! Piss off and play on someone else's gate!' Then we got our own goal. About four doors up from our house there was a small area of waste ground, and the people who lived there had a wall built for them by the council. It didn't take long for us to paint some goalposts up on the wall. Suddenly, we had somewhere where no one would come out and move us along. There'd be an ongoing battle of the goal being rubbed out and us painting it back up again, but we'd be out there playing whenever we got the chance.

It was heaven. We would play until ten or half ten at night, until we had been shouted at a dozen times, told 'This is your *last* warning!' and dragged in by the scruff of our necks. That was the way it was back then: you could play out in the streets until all hours and your parents would not be worried about where you were or what might happen. It wasn't that our families didn't care, they just felt comfortable their children were safe, outside with their mates. These days, parents don't want anything to happen to their children; if it means them not being out once darkness falls, then so be it. I know, with my own children, you are never comfortable when they go out at all.

We didn't just play football on the waste ground. Just down the road from our house was an area called Windy Harbour. Windy Harbour used to be a bit like Hackney Marshes in East London: it was about half a mile long and full of football pitches. As the name suggests, it was somewhat open to the elements. These days, Windy Harbour is the home to Liverpool FC's football academy, but back then it was every man and football mad boy for himself.

My brother and I would go down to Windy Harbour and practise. Later, we would go up there almost every night. I'd say to Ronnie, 'Want to go and have a kick about?' and off we'd go. I'd practise kicking with my left foot because that was my weaker one, and spend hours doing patterns to strengthen it. We'd play 'cross ball': I'd stand on one side of the goal and Ronnie the other, and we'd take turns to try and clip the ball onto the crossbar. It's a great exercise in terms of getting a feel for the ball and learning how to weight your kicks. Those kinds of exercises undoubtedly helped me. If there were other people about, you'd have a game where one person would be the keeper and the other eight to ten are all trying to score a goal: last one to score goes in goal for the next game. I loved Windy Harbour – I knew I could go there and always find someone to kick about with. No matter how bad the weather was, there was always at least one game of football going on.

Sometimes my dad would come down and pass balls to me. Other times, he'd just come and sit and watch. There was a wall at the top end, and he'd come and perch there. He wouldn't say anything, just used to sit there and observe. And then you would turn around again and he would be gone. He just wanted to see what we were doing, and then he'd disappear again. That was my dad all over: very understated.

I was basically a good child when I was growing up. I didn't particularly get into trouble at school or anything like that. Don't get me wrong, I had my mischievous moments, but I never had one proper run in with the police. There were times when we would be out and the police would come over and ask, 'What are you up to lads?' But it never went any further than that. I think I was probably too afraid of my dad to get into any real trouble.

At school, I got detentions for being late and talking in class but never for any fighting or disrupting class. I was your classic 'could do better' kid. I did okay and didn't dislike going to school, except right towards the end. When I was fifteen or sixteen, I just wanted to play football. By that point I knew what I wanted to do and felt as if school was starting to get in the way. That seemed very clear to me: I didn't know whether or not I would become a professional footballer but that was the only thing that mattered to me. Looking back, it was a stupid attitude to have. If things hadn't worked out at Bolton, I wouldn't have had much to fall back on.

It might not surprise you to learn that all my favourite teachers were the ones who took us for sport. Mr Brennan was probably the youngest and the coolest one. He was a good-looking guy, had a big moustache like Tom Selleck and all the girls liked him. He was very sporty and really good with me. He could see I was a decent footballer and he helped me a lot. Then there was Dowie Jones: he was the sort of big teacher that didn't say much, but had the loudest bark. He took us for rugby, and if you didn't want to play it he would grab you by the scruff of the neck and drag you onto the field. He was the teacher everyone was frightened of. He was also the sort of teacher who started to treat you differently as you got older. You could have a proper conversation with him, and by the end I thought he was great. He asked me back to the school after I had left and I really enjoyed seeing him and telling him what I was doing.

My primary school was Simonswood. It was just around the corner from our house, a five-minute walk away. My mum used to work there as a dinner lady. That had its good points and bad points. When it was dinner time, I'd always get my extra chips and extra pudding. But back out in the schoolyard afterwards, my mum would be one of those watching over the children. So she'd be watching me to check I was behaving and I would get it in the neck if I didn't!

It was a lovely little school, and it's such a shame it isn't there any more. A few years ago the school got burnt down: someone broke in and set off a fire. The school wasn't restored, but ended up getting amalgamated with another school in the area. It's really sad, because you have your memories as a child and your associations with that place. I drive past the site now, and it hasn't been developed. It's just there, empty, with its overgrown weeds. To think that you spent six or seven happy years of your childhood there, and it's now just left there, in this condition. It's sad.

From there I went on to Ruffwood Comprehensive. That was the daunting one for me. It was a big school, with a lot of pupils and a reputation. Like Simonswood, it also doesn't exist any more: the government labelled it a failing school and it was closed and merged with another comprehensive. Certainly, when I was there, it wasn't a good place to be if you were quiet. The school had its fair share of bullies, and you had lads who would find their targets and pick on them relentlessly. I'd always been quite a small child, but fortunately for me I had this growth spurt when I was thirteen or fourteen, so wasn't usually picked on.

Even so, they'd still test you out. One of the hot spots was always the dinner queue, where the bigger lads would barge in front of you, and see what you were going to do about it. I had a few confrontations like that. I remember one time, one of the toughest kids in the school, a real hard lad, decided to push in front of me. On this occasion, I wasn't having it, and told him to get back down the queue. There was a bit of a scuffle and he said he'd sort me out after school. I was left thinking, what have I done? I've pissed off one of the hardest kids in the school, and he's going to deck me. All that afternoon, I was thinking, what should I do? Should I wait for him and stand up for myself, or make a run for it as soon as the bell went? I decided to wait, and luckily nothing came of it. After that, this lad was all right with me. I think he respected that I'd stood up to him.

That was typical of the school: yes, you'd get tested, but as long as you stood up for yourself, then you'd be okay. It probably didn't hurt either that I was good at football. That went a long way in the playground. It meant that the hard lads always wanted you to be on their team. You'd get to know them a bit, and they'd be a bit more friendly towards you. The more people knew about my football, the less confrontations I got involved in. There'd still be scuffles in the games, people trying it on, but as I got bigger, that happened less and less. I had my mates, decent kids, and we didn't go looking for trouble.

Although I enjoyed all sport, it was always football that I was really into. We played rugby union for about two years, by which point they realised that I wasn't going to be a rugby player. So they let me off the hook with the rugby and allowed me to focus on the football, which I was thrilled to bits about. That was by far what I was best at. When I had been younger, I hadn't been bad at cross country, but as I grew I lost my speed. That was a process that continued when I became a professional footballer: I wasn't slow, but I was never what you'd call quick, not physically anyway. For me, my speed was all in my mind, on reading situations.

I played for the school team: we were okay and had a couple of decent players. I played all over. Sometimes I was out wide, sometimes in midfield, and other times I was up front. It was all a bit like the football scene in *Kes*, if you remember that, with Brian Glover bossing the boys about. The teacher would tell someone they were playing in defence and they'd say, 'I don't like playing there'.

'Well, you're playing there today.'

'But I don't want to. Can I play in midfield instead?'

'Okay, you can play there today. Stubbs, you're going at the back.'

'But sir, can't I play up front . . .'

And on it would go. The only bit missing from *Kes* was the teacher playing centre-forward himself! I've always liked that film, and thought it captured exactly what school days at the time were like. We'd chuck our kit all over the changing rooms and get bollocked for that ('Get that kit off the floor right now!'). We'd get shouted at to clean our boots. And we used to get a clip round the ear if we misbehaved, Brian Clough style. Teachers were more hands-on in those days. If you were ordered off the pitch and they thought you were leaving too slowly, you could expect to be grabbed by the scruff of the neck and dragged off. You wouldn't be able to get away with that now. The strange thing is, even though the teachers did that to us, we probably had more respect for them than the young kids do today.

The best players from the school would go on to be picked for Kirkby Boys, which was a team made up of the best players from the area. Historically, Kirkby Boys had always been a strong team: they were up there with the likes of Sefton, Huyton and Liverpool Boys. Steven Gerrard played for Huyton when he was growing up; when I was playing, the Liverpool Boys team featured the likes of Steve McManaman, and later on Wayne Rooney played for them. So it was an honour when I was chosen to play for Kirkby.

The first team I played for was when I was about eight or nine, and that was Pingwood FC. That's where it all started for me. I went from playing on the street and kickabouts at Windy Harbour to going to Pingwood for a trial game and getting in the team. Pingwood was probably the best team in the area. The manager at the time, a guy called Josh Godfrey who is sadly no longer with us, had a reputation for finding the best players to play for Pingwood. As a result, the club won quite a lot of things. The kids team that I was in was very successful: we won a whole trophy cabinet full of leagues and cups.

Pingwood FC was so called because there was a local pub of the same name: a lot of the local names ended in 'wood' because the area was originally all woodland, before it was cleared to make way for houses. There was a pitch outside the pub and that was where we'd play our home games. Pingwood had a few teams but didn't go all the way up in terms of age range. I think eleven- or twelve-year-olds were the oldest teams. That was quite common back then, simply because people couldn't afford to run a whole group of teams. These days, if you play for one of these teams you usually pay subs – however many pounds a week. Back then, the money would come out of the manager's pocket, or in our case, the pub. We never paid to play, the only exception being when we were travelling a long distance for a competition.

Because Pingwood's pitch was right outside the pub, we used to get changed inside and come out and play. Sometimes if we had an early kick-off on a Sunday, the pub was still locked up from having a late one the night before. Then we'd have to get changed outside in the freezing cold. After the match, everyone would go back to the pub. The parents would have a pint, and some would have several. We'd be allowed in, and would sit quietly in the corner until it was time to go home.

I played striker for Pingwood. That might seem a bit strange for someone who ended up making a career as a centre-half, but that's partly because the best footballer in the team ended up at the front. It was also partly because as a child – and this is no different now – everyone wants to be the focus, everyone wants to be the centre-forward. Every boy having a kick about in the street wants to be the one who scores that winning goal. Whether you ultimately end up a striker, defender or midfield player, you still want to be the person who shoots the ball into the top corner, the person wheeling away and doing the celebration.

At the time I was small and quick, and those sort of players usually ended up playing up front. As a striker, I scored all types of goals. My right foot is naturally my better foot, but my left was good, too, and I always made sure to practise with that as much as my right down at Windy Harbour. So I'd score with both feet: shots and tap-ins, headers too, the lot. Then, as I started to grow, I began the process of working my way back through the team, from striker to left wing, to midfield and then from midfield to the centre of defence. It was a good job I stopped where I did, because I was never going to be a decent goalkeeper!

It was when I dropped back from being a striker to a midfielder that my understanding of the game really improved. That turned out to be invaluable when I became a centre-half. There's a saying we have in football – 'quick and thick' – by which we mean that players who have a bit of pace about them can sometimes end up getting a bit lazy. They can rely on their speed to get them out of situations, so they don't have to think about and read the game like others do. As I grew and dropped back into midfield, my game became less about pace and more about being one or two steps ahead of the opposition players. My feet might not have been the quickest on the pitch, but my mind was always up there. I learnt to read the game, taught myself to spot what was going to happen and made sure I was in the right place before it did. The understanding I gained at that early age was one of the reasons I was ultimately able to play at the top of my profession.

The routine at Pingwood was that there'd be a practice session once a week and then matches on a Saturday and a Sunday. The training sessions would be down by the pub and I really enjoyed them – there'd be a mixture of small games, and then a big one to finish with. The matches themselves would be about twenty minutes each way. There'd be your classic pieces of orange at half-time, and blackcurrant or orange juice on a special occasion. No sports or energy drinks back in those days!

I enjoyed playing for Pingwood, and especially for Josh. As a manager, Josh was a brilliant guy. He had a really warm personality, and was great with kids, always very encouraging. Even if you didn't play well it was, 'Ah well, don't worry about it. There is always next week.' If you did have a decent game, Josh would be 'How good were you today?' and you'd go home feeling six inches taller. Ask anyone who played for him what he was like, and thirty years on, they'd all tell you what a lovely guy he was.

I was about eight or nine when I first started playing for Pingwood, which these days would seem quite old. Now, the kids start that bit younger: five or six is the norm. That is the way it has gone: they have barely managed to walk properly and they start to kick a ball. For me, that's wrong. At the same time I know that if a club like Everton didn't do it, then someone else would do it. And before you know it, you're starting to fall behind as a club.

Even so, part of me still thinks you have got to let children be children. You have got to let them enjoy their childhood because

once that time is gone, it's gone forever. I know as a child I bene-
fited from having that freedom (or at least, I had freedom within
the rules that my dad gave me!). I knew what was right and what
was wrong; I knew how far I could go. There's a danger with footballers starting too young that they can end up a little zombie-like
on the pitch, especially when their parents are shouting instructions from the touchline. I cringe, I actually physically cringe
when I see what the parents of today are putting their children
through. Football has gone to a level no one ever dreamt of, in
terms of the money on offer for the top players. The kids have still
got dreams of just being a footballer, just like my generation did,
but now I think the parents' dreams have taken over from their
children. You come across parents who are using them almost as
guinea pigs; they see their kids as their golden ticket for a better
life in the future.

I'm grateful that my parents supported me in my football, but
never in that way. My dad would come and watch every match:
whatever the weather, however long it took to get to the ground,
he'd be there. Sometimes my mum would be there too: she
wouldn't always know what was going on, but she'd turn up to
offer her support. Dad would not have been one of those parents
who shout and scream from the touchline. He wouldn't say a
word, but just let me play. He'd give me encouragement but that
was as far as it went. Don't get me wrong, it wasn't that he didn't
have an opinion, but he would save it until after the game. If I
played well, he'd say, 'You did really good today'. If I hadn't, he
wouldn't say anything. That silence after the game was enough
for me to know that I hadn't performed.

It's not just the age that we start our young players that has
become an issue in recent years. The question of how we coach
them has also become a live issue. There's an ongoing debate
between the continental approach, which is geared towards

smaller games and more practice with the ball, and the traditional British system that favours competitive, full-size games at an earlier age. There is a move to try and get more contact time with young players: in Spain, Germany, France and Italy they have a curriculum which is geared on a number of hours of coaching. Someone's worked out the numbers, and in Britain we have the least contact time with the players in terms of coaching.

I don't think our climate does us any favours: in somewhere like Spain, they can be out on the pitch all day. In this country, you never quite know what the summer has in store, and then you've got an autumn and winter where you probably do know what you are going to get – and it's only worse. So that's less time we have with the players before we even start. But where else are we going wrong? Is it because our coaches aren't good enough? Is it because we don't work enough technically with the players? Is it down to the physicality of the players we are choosing? – it's noticeable that Spain is one of the smallest teams in world football.

I think we have got some fantastic coaches in England. But when you look at how countries like Spain coach from an early age, it is definitely different to the way we do things here. I think we need to look at the way our teams coach their young players technically. We can't keep producing players, come up against the likes of Brazil, Argentina, Spain, and France, and find ourselves saying, 'Technically their players are better than us'. That can't just be down to physics or the way we are built – it has got to be down to the culture.

Individually, are the Spanish or Argentinian players better than those we have got in the England team? For me, you have to say no. Are Iniesta or Xavi better than, say, Steven Gerrard or Wayne Rooney? Gerrard, I think, is one of the best players that this country has produced. Wayne Rooney is probably the best talent we have had in this country for years: for all the claims that Spanish players are 'technically better', Wayne is a footballer who is technically exceptional.

The difference is not in the players themselves, but how they come together as a team. For whatever reason, Spain understands how to do this, whereas I don't think England play as a team. Is that because of egos? Is it because of money? Is it because they have not got the right blend – is the person picking the team not getting it right? It's odd, because it should almost be the other way round. If young English players are spending more time playing matches as a team and the Spanish players are having more contact time with the coaches, they should be the ones individually focused and the England players less technical but better as a unit.

I do think our coaching is catching up. The training facilities that we have got now in this country are first rate, better than they ever have been. Whereas my generation could complain that the pitch was rubbish, or the training facilities were poor, or come up with any number of reasons, now the facilities for a young player are superb. From an academy point of view, they have got the best pitches and the best facilities that you could ever dream of. There are gyms, sports scientists, nutritionists, there's yoga – in all, a wealth of experts and knowledge to learn from.

Are we producing players to replicate the quality of these facilities? At the moment, I have to say no. That comes down to a lot of things but the main two from my point of view have always been the scouting and the culture. You can look at a number of other factors but if your scouting is not right and your culture is not right, you are never going to get close to bridging that coaching gap. And I think that is what needs to be addressed more than anything.

So I do think that smaller pitches and smaller games can help. In Spain they play more of these sorts of games. Fewer players means you get more touches; smaller pitches means you have to learn to control it better, pass it better, be smarter with your turns and tricks. The result is that the players have a better understanding of the game, and this is noticeable as the players get older. Technically, as I say, I don't think the players are better. But their understanding often is.

Our coaching courses here have always been fairly forward thinking. One of the things that you do when you study for your coaching badges in this country is to look at different cultures. As part of the course I did, we went to Denmark to watch the Under-21 European Championships. We spent ten days there and studied the matches and styles intensively. We did an exchange programme with UEFA and spent time in Switzerland at their headquarters in Nyon, along with coaches from the Czech Republic, Poland and other countries. All the time we were swapping views and exchanging ideas on football and training cultures. That's an important part of getting your coaching badges, and the course encourages you to be receptive to new ideas. It may take a while, but that will all feed through into the coaching culture here.

Going back to my own childhood and practising all those hours with my weaker foot, that's something I worry you don't see as much of these days in this country. You very rarely see players who will get a bag of balls and go off by themselves. I still remember how Wayne Rooney was a breath of fresh air when he first came up as a sixteen-year-old, to train with the Everton first team. Wayne would be the one who would be the first out on the training pitch. He would be out there about ten to ten with a bag of balls, ready for training at half ten. He would be kicking balls from the halfway line, or having shots at the goal, trying to put them in the top corner. After training, too, he would be working on all areas of his game: left foot, left foot finishing, movements in and around the box, and heading. Wayne was not great at heading to start with; it was probably one of the weakest parts of his game, but he set himself to work to get that sorted out.

It always surprises me you don't see that more often. I think maybe what has happened is that it's a by-product of young footballers having too much done for them. Sometimes, it feels as though we have got to the stage where the only things we are not doing for the young players is wiping their arses. The days of young players cleaning the first team's boots, cleaning the first-team dressing rooms and so on has gone. That's a shame, I think. As a young player growing up, that could be my highlight of the week: on a Monday morning, if the player had had a good game or scored a goal, he would come up to you and say, 'Stubbsy, well done. My boots were gleaming on Saturday, here's a tenner. Make sure they are like that next week.' And it was like, *My god, clean – get in there*. I used to love it. I was there after training, scrubbing and cleaning.

That work ethic has disappeared from young footballers over the last decade or so. You wonder why players can't work it out for themselves on the pitch, and it's because the clubs have taken it upon themselves to do everything for them. You might ask why clubs are doing that, but I think it's because of the mentality of young players coming through. It's what they've come to expect. That's unlikely to change because it's harder to find good British players these days: I'd say that was the general consensus across the board. It's not rocket science to work out why: we are in the age of the Xbox, social media and the Internet. You don't have a generation of kids on the street corner playing football: they're inside staring at a computer screen. That reduces the talent pool available so when you find someone who is talented, you stick to them like glue. You give them what they want, even if that isn't what they really need.

\*     \*     \*

I'd been playing for Pingwood for a couple of years when I was scouted. I was eleven at the time, in my last year at junior school. I didn't know I was being watched. Back then, scouts would just be in normal civvy clothes; unlike today, where they turn up in these enormous coats with the club badge on, making it obvious they're from Liverpool or Man United or whoever. I'm never quite sure if that's useful. It means that everyone knows which clubs are watching which players; it also means the players know they're being watched, and that can be quite intimidating.

In my case, I didn't know the scout had been there. I'd just be focusing on the game. During the match, he'd asked around to find out who my father was, and went to talk to him. At the end of the game, Dad was waiting for me with a big grin on his face.

'The scout from Everton was here, son,' he said. 'They want you to go in and do some training with them.'

I didn't believe him at first. 'Come on,' I said, 'you must be joking.'

'It's true,' my dad persisted. 'They want you to go up next Thursday.'

The feeling was amazing. I was like, *wow.* To have been scouted, and not just by anyone but my own team, Everton. I was absolutely thrilled, and also quite nervous, especially as the Thursday came round. It felt like a big chance, and I really didn't want to blow it. I came home from school that day, and Dad was waiting for me to take the bus there together. He'd bought me a new Everton football kit, so I got changed into that, put my boots into a bag and we set off. We got the bus to West Derby and walked up to Bellefield, which was where Everton were training at the time.

I trained with the other boys. I was new and they'd been there a while, which didn't help with the nerves, but I did my best to fit in. I didn't get taken on immediately after that first trial; it was only three or four weeks later that Dad and I were called in for a meeting.

'We like what we have seen,' I was told, just the news I'd been dreaming to hear. 'We'd like you to sign for us.'

As a boyhood Evertonian, it felt like a dream come true. In my imagination, I could see my progression to playing for the first team laid out before me. Little did I realise then, but it would be a near two-decade journey before I finally made that debut.

# 3

## From YTS to the Big Time

Growing up in Liverpool, you were either a blue or a red. For me, it was obvious what colour scarf I was going to put on. My dad had always been an Evertonian, as indeed had all the family (Kirkby itself was split, with a mixture of Everton and Liverpool fans; the playground at school was always full of both). Dad wasn't a season ticket holder – he couldn't afford one – but we'd get tickets whenever we could, and if someone else had a spare, we'd take that. Even if I couldn't go, we would be in on a Saturday afternoon listening to the radio. We'd crowd round a little transistor listening to the commentary on the game and watching the scores come in on the telly: Dickie Davies on ITV's *World of Sport*. Then in the evening, we watched *Match of the Day*. Because my brothers and sisters were older, they'd often be out on a Saturday night, so it would just be the three of us: me, Mum and Dad. We'd have sweets and cocoa, and settle down to watch.

So being taken on by Everton Boys was simply the best thing that had ever happened to me. When I was younger I used to go to Bellefield and stand at the edge of the gateway, waiting for the players to come out and get photographs. That is what we'd do during the school holidays: hang around the gates. My mates and I would get the bus down and there'd be a whole group of us waiting – then I'd run home and tell my dad who I'd seen.

Now I was through the gate, on the other side. I'd train after school, and it would be quite a tight schedule – one session after another for an hour or so, from 4.30 until 8.30. I'd play a match for Everton at the weekend, but would also still be allowed to turn out for Pingwood – the club were happy for you still to play for another team. You'd just have to strike a balance between the two.

When I first went to Everton, I played on the left side of midfield. I loved the training at Bellefield: we used to work on technical skills, lots of exercises to improve dribbling, passing and turning. We'd play various small-sided games, and then usually a big one to finish. All the while, I kept my eye out for the first-team players. They'd usually finished their training by the time we turned up, but sometimes you'd see the last ones leaving, or maybe spy a player in for afternoon treatment. There'd be a little ripple among the boys – 'Look who's over there!' – and a clamour to see who it was. The players I kept a particular eye out for were Peter Reid and Graeme Sharp: they were my main heroes. Adrian Heath was another favourite, so much so that I got my hair cut like his, a tight perm, which was all the rage at the time.

It's funny looking back: I was always chasing after Peter Reid with my autograph book. Peter was a typical Scouser – 'Yep, no problem'. He was great with me then, and exactly the same years later when he heard I'd been diagnosed with cancer. He was straight on the phone, no messing about, telling me that I was a Scouser and a fighter and that I was going to be okay. It was a great boost at the time, and I really appreciated him still looking out for me.

There was no payment at the time for being an Everton Boy. That's still the case today, I think – though help can come in the form of expenses. But we did get tickets to go and see matches at Goodison, which was a great perk. Everton were one of the best teams in the land in the mid-eighties, and match tickets could be like gold dust.

The first time I went to see Everton play I was about eight, and I fell in love with Goodison Park from my first visit. I'd stand with my dad at the Gwladys Street End. The way the terraces were set up was that there were the old metal barriers all spaced out evenly, leading down to a brick wall at the front. They'd put crates down the front for the young ones who weren't tall enough to see over the wall. That was where I first watched them, on a crate looking over the wall. It was magical: the best view in the house. As I got older, I'd stand further back with my dad, sometimes sitting on one of the metal bars. The best moments would be when Everton scored and everyone rushed forwards in delight. There'd be this mad rush down the front, squeezing and squashing you as everyone cheered and clapped. Then everyone would shuffle back, and the game would go on.

I can't remember exactly my first match at Goodison as a spectator, but it would have been right at the end of the seventies, when Gordon Lee was in charge. I watched the team during the tail end of his tenure, before Howard Kendall took over in 1981. I was lucky: it was the perfect time to grow up as an Everton fan, given the success that his team would go on to achieve.

Dad would tell me all about the Everton teams of the past. He'd talk about the championship winning team of the sixties, about famous players like Dixie Dean, Alex Young and Dave Hickson. I remember it went a bit over my head: he'd tell me how Dave Hickson was a big hard player, but it's difficult to get an idea of someone when you haven't seen them play yourself.

At the time I was growing up and getting into football – aged seven, eight, nine – Liverpool were hugely successful as a football club, and were one of the dominant teams in the whole of Europe. I suppose that apart from the mid-eighties in my memory and previous great sides through the decades, Everton have often found themselves playing second fiddle to Liverpool. By which I mean that we have had our successes, and some amazing ones – nine league championships, five FA Cups – but the club has never enjoyed continued, sustained success over a period of years in the way that Liverpool had in the seventies and eighties. That has probably been the hardest thing for Everton fans over the years. Because I was young when I got into football, I was quite happy that many of those Liverpool success stories seemed to pass me by quite quickly. I only started to take notice and worry about Liverpool when I was ten, eleven, twelve. That's when I started to go to games week in, week out, and, luckily enough, that was the time when Everton started to become really successful.

I always wanted Liverpool to lose. Even if it was a European final, I'd still want the other team to win: unfortunately, that seldom happened at the time! I may not have been a fan of the Reds, but that didn't stop me having a huge amount of respect for some of their players. Alan Hansen, in particular, was someone I admired hugely. He was always so elegant on the ball, and when I found my own position in the team moving back towards defence, he was the player I used to watch, and wanted to emulate.

By the mid-eighties, Howard Kendall had turned Everton into one of the top sides in the country: Everton won the FA Cup in 1984, beating Watford in the final, and the following year went on to win the league and the Cup Winners' Cup. By this point, I was getting tickets for pretty much every home game. I didn't go to the 1984 FA Cup final, unfortunately; my first experience of Wembley came at the following year's FA Cup final, when Everton lost to Manchester United. My second experience of Wembley wasn't much better, when Everton got to the final again the following year, this time to lose to Liverpool.

What I do remember strongly from the 1984 Cup final was the open top bus parade after Everton had beaten Watford. That was a magical moment. My dad, my brother and I went down for that, all done up in our Everton scarves and hats. The roads were all cordoned off to traffic and filled with Everton fans. All the terrace songs were being bellowed and the crowds were so deep you could hardly see the bus. We'd get a glimpse then run a hundred yards down the road in the hope of seeing it again.

There's no doubt that Howard put together a fantastic team. To win the FA Cup, the European Cup Winners' Cup and the league twice in three years takes some doing. What was a shame was that because of the ban on English clubs in Europe following Heysel in 1985, that Everton team never got their chance to show what they could do in the European Cup. There's no doubt in my mind that had they had the chance to compete, they'd have been right up there, among the best clubs in Europe. You only had to look at some of their results on the way to winning the Cup Winners' Cup the previous season to see that – coming from behind to beat Bayern Munich 3–1 in the semi-final, for example.

There was anger among Everton fans over the consequences of Heysel. The fans felt harshly done by for not being allowed to compete in Europe. That anger wasn't aimed at Liverpool: it was more about UEFA and their decision to impose a blanket ban. It was UEFA who made that strong stance to ban English clubs from European competitions. The result for Everton was that rather than the team getting stronger, it started instead to splinter. Howard Kendall, who by the way I don't think I've ever heard an ex-player have a bad word to say about, left to go to Athletic

Bilbao. Gary Lineker, who'd joined the club from Leicester City to help us win the league in 1985–86, went off to play for Barcelona. If Everton had been able to offer them European football, things might have been different.

Then, at the end of the eighties, there was Hillsborough. Such was the magnitude of the events that the fact that Liverpool were our rivals was neither here nor there. I remember feeling physically sick on the day, when I heard what had happened. I think that anyone who'd stood on a terrace had a 'there but for the grace of God' feeling that day. The Liverpool fans had all sorts of accusations thrown at them over the events of that afternoon, with the police and the politicians all hiding from the facts and covering their arses over what really happened. But the fans knew. Liverpool as a city knew. When the *Sun* printed its front page accusations about what Liverpool fans had done, under the heading 'The Truth', sales of the newspaper on Merseyside sank overnight: red or blue, everyone in Liverpool boycotted it.

The press allegations about the fans were both disgusting and false. The truth – the real truth – would take years to finally come out. It took the relatives of those who died years to get the justice they deserved. To see the huge relief, anger and satisfaction from that . . . I sat there watching the telly and shaking my head thinking, I can't believe what I am listening to. What these people had been put through for so many years by what were basically a bunch of cowards. For it to have gone on for so many years, without anyone saying anything, was not right. There is no place for it in society.

The result of Hillsborough was the Taylor Report and the introduction of all-seater stadiums. Looking back to my childhood years as a fan, it's difficult not to be nostalgic for the days of terracing. When I started getting tickets from being part of the academy, these would be seats up in the top balcony. They were so high it felt like you were in the clouds: so steep that you didn't want to lean forwards in case you fell! You'd get a different perspective up there, not just the view of the game, but also the rest of the crowd. I'd look down at the Gwladys Street End, where I used to stand, with more than a little bit of envy: you'd watch the celebrating and hardcore singing, and part of you wished you were down there among it.

When the terracing went, so inevitably did a bit of that atmosphere. Not completely, of course: Goodison is fortunate that it has been able to maintain its character as a football venue. It's still an old ground, with the fans so close to the pitch they can almost feel on top of you. Speak to any opposition team and they'll tell you how much they don't like coming to Everton to play: it's such a hostile place for an away player. The Goodison crowd undoubtedly gives the home team a lift: there's a common football cliché about the fans being like a twelfth man, but Goodison is one of those places where it's actually true. The flipside of having the fans on top of you is that they're right on your back when you're not doing well. The Everton fans have always been a fair crowd, and as long as you are trying, they'll accept that. But anyone who isn't putting a shift in can expect to get it.

If becoming an Everton Boy was one of the best moments in my life, then one of my worst was to follow a couple of years later. At the end of each season, you'd get to sit down with the academy manager. He'd talk through your performances and the progress that you'd made. The first couple of years I had these meetings, I sailed through. The third year, when I was fourteen, the situation was different. I went for the meeting and the academy manager said that there was only one place for the following season available, and I was one of two players they were going to have to choose between for it.

'I'm sorry Alan,' the academy manager said. 'We've decided to go with the other guy.'

I was heartbroken. As soon as I'd put that Everton kit on and had started going there week in, week out to train, I'd assumed this was it: I was on the first steps to becoming a professional football player with my boyhood club. Now I felt as if my dream had been shattered into a million pieces. That was it. The end. The future I'd been planning for myself had been taken away. If I wasn't going to become an Everton footballer, I simply had no idea what I'd do with my life instead.

Now I'm on the other side, I know what a tough call that is for the coach to make. But that's what you're paid to do: to make those sort of decisions. You are going to get some wrong, unfortunately, but you like to think you get the majority of them right. In my case, they simply thought the other guy at that age was the better player. It was irrelevant, really, that he didn't go on to be anything. Different players develop at different ages – I certainly wasn't the first player to be let go to make it elsewhere, and won't be the last either. At Everton alone, two other high-profile players who were subsequently let go were Leighton Baines and Phil Jagielka. I didn't have any hard feelings towards those making the call and I'm sure Bainesy and Jags don't either – hence the fact we all returned, when given the chance.

Of course, I wasn't quite as forgiving as this at the time. How could I be? I felt as though the wind had been taken out of my sails. What made it worse was that I simply hadn't had an inkling it was coming; that was probably one of the reasons it knocked me so hard. But there was no comeback. I gathered my stuff and made my way to the bus stop to head home. Dad was there and tried to talk sense in to me. Don't worry about it, he told me: it is not the end of the world, we'll go somewhere else. He must have said a hundred things to me as we waited for the bus, but I couldn't remember a single one of them. I was away in a world of my own.

I cried as we sat there. Dad put his arm round me and said, 'It's all right son.' He said that it was just an opinion, that they'd had to make a choice, that it wasn't anything about me as a player.

'It's up to you to prove them wrong,' he said. 'You need to get out there and show them they've made a mistake.'

He was right, of course. The rejection, as rejections sometimes do, only served to make me stronger. It put fire in my belly and spurred me on to succeed elsewhere. Sitting at the cold bus stop, however, such success still felt a long way away.

As it happened, I didn't have to wait long at all for a call to come. Within a couple of weeks of being let go by Everton, I was approached after playing a match for Kirkby Boys. The guy introduced himself as a scout for Bolton Wanderers and explained that that they had been watching me. Would I be interested in coming and talking about playing for them?

Bolton in the mid-eighties were doing as badly as Everton were doing well. They were bumping along the bottom of what was then the Third Division (League One in today's money) and at the end of the 1986–87 season would be relegated into football's bottom tier. But they were a club with a fantastic history and heritage, and it felt an exciting opportunity. Being taken on by them kept my dream of becoming a professional footballer alive.

Getting from Liverpool to Bolton without a car was easier said than done. Fortunately, there were a few lads from Liverpool going over and so we were able to travel together. I'd get a bus from Kirkby to Heyton, where I'd meet up with the others outside a pub. One of the other boys was a kid called Ronnie Taylor, and his parents had a minibus. We would give him some money for taking us up there, to cover the cost of his diesel.

Going to school in Liverpool and training at Bolton in the evening was quite a tight schedule. I'd get home from school, have a quick bite to eat and then I would have to leave and start my journey to Bolton by four o'clock. I'd get the bus to Heyton for about quarter to five, the minibus would leave about five and we'd get to Bolton for six. We'd train for an hour and a half and then head home. I wouldn't be back until about half nine or ten. And I'd do that twice a week, every Tuesday and Thursday.

The Bolton academy was situated round the back of Burnden Park, where Bolton played before the Reebok Stadium was built. The facilities weren't quite those of a modern Premier League club: it was basically a square of Astroturf, about sixty metres by forty, with a cage around it. The shrunken size wasn't a hindrance, though: it meant the games were small and the training was good from a technical point of view. In terms of growing as a footballer, the intensity of those sessions was invaluable.

I quickly settled into the routine: training two nights during the week, Goodison to watch Everton on a Saturday and playing for Bolton on a Sunday. Even though Everton had let me go as a player, that never affected how I felt about the club or changed my relationship as a fan. They were still my team, and always would be.

The Christmas after I was fifteen, I was called in by Bolton for a meeting about my future. Uh-oh, I thought, after the experience at Everton. This time round, though, it was good news. They asked my dad in as well, and told us that they wanted to offer me a scholarship. This was a two-year apprenticeship, what in those days was called a YTS placement or Youth Training Scheme. I was over the moon, to borrow a football cliché of the time. Seriously, this felt like the moment that I was starting to make that step up: the pieces in the jigsaw to becoming a professional footballer were falling in to place.

The YTS placement was set to begin after I'd done my exams at sixteen. Because I knew I had my place, it was a killer in terms of motivating me to do any revision. I didn't put any effort in at all, which was silly of me looking back. I wasn't stupid or bad at school – I was probably above average when I applied myself. But apply myself was something I didn't do, and the results I got reflected that. Looking back, it was a risky thing to do: if the football career hadn't taken off, I'd have had little to fall back on. It's certainly not a course of action I'd recommend to the young players I work with today.

Not that I was thinking like that as I started my YTS. I was now doing football full time, and couldn't have been happier. It was fortunate I loved what I was doing, because YTS pay wasn't the highest in the world: I got the princely sum of £29.50 a week plus expenses which wasn't much even back then. I used to get the train over – you could get a train from Kirkby to Wigan, and then on from Wigan to Bolton. There were a few of us who got on at Kirkby, and there'd always be a fight to see who could get in the toilet, lock themselves in and therefore avoid paying. You could squeeze two in, and we'd hide in there and tell anyone who knocked on the door that we were feeling sick. There weren't any barriers at Bolton, so when the train pulled in, we'd open the door, look to see if the guard was about, and then make a run for it. All of which sounds quite childish, but our expenses were £65 a week, so if you could avoid the train fare, that was another £15 or so you were getting.

Doing the YTS definitely felt like a step up. In terms of my football, I was playing for the youth team, so you were up against older players, and that was definitely a test. We had coaching every day. We'd train in the morning, from 10.30 until lunchtime, then we'd break, train again after lunch until about two, and then do our jobs until it was time to go home, at about 4.30.

The list of jobs the YTS lads were given to do sometimes seemed never-ending: we'd be given all the boots to clean; there was an Astroturf carpet in the corridor, which had to be brushed and swept every day; we had to sweep the terraces on a Monday morning after a game; we painted the stands; and one of the lads would have to wash the manager's car.

We also had to clean the dressing rooms. That was a job and a half. We'd mop and brush the floor, move all the kit away, scrub the baths, the showerheads and the toilets. We used Vim powder to wash the baths: you'd wet them first, these big old fashioned baths, then sprinkle the Vim, scrub around and wash it off. There would probably be three of us cleaning the bath, another couple doing the showers, three doing the home dressing room, the same doing the away dressing room.

The next day, when the senior players came in, they would run their fingers along the surface of the baths. If you hadn't washed all the Vim off, it would leave a dust behind. If the players found traces of Vim, you had to do a forfeit there and then in the dressing room. Forfeits came in a number of different ways: you might get roughed up, be given a few slaps and punches; you might have to strip to your pants and get covered in boot polish or liniment; or you'd be made to stand there, your body covered, and sing them a song, usually something humiliating like a nursery rhyme.

That sort of thing probably wouldn't be allowed nowadays, but it was all part of team building and growing up. And in its brutal way, it worked. We had real respect for the senior players as a result: we had to knock before we were allowed in the first-team rooms, and could only enter if someone invited us in. It meant we looked up to them, and it instilled in us a real sense of pride in the place.

There was much, of course, to be proud about. Bolton had been one of the original members of the Football League back in

1888. They'd won the FA Cup three times in the 1920s, including the first final held at Wembley Stadium. They'd won it again in the 1950s, when Nat Lofthouse was the team's star player. When I first joined, these glory days seemed a long time past. The club were down in the lower divisions and part of the ground had been sold off to the Co-op as a supermarket, in order to raise money. But the expectation of the fans, and desire to drive the team back up the divisions, was undimmed.

The manager when I started doing the YTS was Phil Neal. He was there until 1992, when Bruce Rioch took over. Phil was someone who came with a wealth of playing experience, winning numerous championships and European titles with Liverpool. He also had a policy at Bolton of promoting youth, which for a young lad like me was great. At one point, his first-team squad of 25 had 17 players under the age of 26, and nine players who had come through the youth system. So I knew, right from the off, that I had a good chance of progressing through the ranks. It was this blend of youth and experience that Bruce would take on to success in the early nineties, the young Bolton side that everyone knows with the likes of Jason McAteer, Alan Thompson, John McGinlay and myself.

I played for the youth team but also for the reserves during this period. That was when I played centre-half for the first time. They were short because of injuries and so I was drafted in to make up the numbers. I wasn't sure how I'd done, but I obviously did okay, because I was picked to play there again. That was my positional journey complete – from playing up front at Pingwood to playing at the back for Bolton. I still played midfield from time to time for Bolton, even when I went up to the first team, but to all intents and purposes, I was a central defender now.

I grew into the position very quickly: it immediately felt a natural fit for me. Sometimes you can be given a position to play and really don't like it, but that wasn't the case with me. I was quite open-minded about being asked to play there and didn't mind when they asked me to play there again. I made mistakes to start with, that's for sure! Part of the learning process was that although I was at the back, I still wanted to play; I didn't want to just hoof and head the ball away but take it out from the back and pass the ball out.

The YTS contract lasted two years, and just after Christmas of the second year, I was told to see the manager. It was at the end of training when I got the message, and I went off to knock nervously on Phil's door.

'We're really happy the way things have gone,' he told me. 'You've done great, so what we'd like to do is offer you a professional contract.'

I had to hold it together, but inside, I was like, *yes!* I'd achieved exactly what I'd set out to do, to become a professional footballer. I had no agent or anything like that: the contract was for £125 a week, Phil said they'd get the contract drawn up, and that was that. That evening, I couldn't get home quick enough to tell my parents. They were thrilled and my dad was chuffed to bits. He knew from having taken me to years of training and sat through watching me play in endless matches just what it meant to me. I was chuffed for him too: it made all his support worthwhile.

The first thing I said once I told them the news was, 'Can I have a new pair of football boots?' I'd worn different makes growing up – my first pair were Patrick Keegans, the ones with two orange and white lines down the back. Then it had been Puma Kings and Nike boots. But the ones I had always wanted, right from a young age, was a pair of Adidas World Cup boots. As far as I was concerned, they were the best. Dad said yes, and the next week I went out and bought myself a pair. I tried them on in the shop and really felt like I'd made it.

It was a good time in my life. It might seem odd to ask my dad's permission to buy the boots, but I was still living at home at this point, and would do so for another few years. I started dating Mandy during this period. I met her at Kirkby Town, a local nightclub one New Year's Eve and we hit it off straightaway. It was quite a night: I had a match to play the following day and what with all the New Year's celebrations, I didn't get to bed until five in the morning. Fortunately, some of the other players had bigger hangovers than I did, so I managed to stay under the manager's radar that afternoon!

All of which made Dad fret a bit. He was worried about the effect on my football, that I'd get distracted. He didn't say anything but you would know. He'd give you one of those looks of his. But I was getting towards that stage then when I was becoming independent. I was beginning to have my own opinions and knew what I wanted. I passed my driving test and got my first car. It was a white Ford Orion 1.4LX, which gave me a bit more freedom. And then at about 20 or 21, Mandy and I moved in together. My dad, I'm sure, was worried about losing his son, but it was never anything like that. It was about me making the break, and setting up on my own.

# 4

---

# Bolton and Bruce

When I went up to the first team, the pros couldn't have been friendlier or more helpful. Phil Brown was the captain at the time, and he was great with me. He was a character for sure, even back then, but a decent player too. Phil had the same suntan as he does now, he always liked to go off and top it up. His dress sense was loud and he'd often come in wearing really wacky shirts, usually with a pair of white trousers. He liked his clothes and thought he was really stylish.

On the pitch, he was a good captain: a shouter and a motivator. He'd be talking away at you the whole game. Phil played at right-back, and to start with I played on the right side of the central pairing, so he was right next to me on the pitch. I say right next to me: he was one of those defenders who'd bomb forward given a chance, and so half the time I ended up covering for him! That first season when I broke into the first team, Phil had a side-bet with me: he bet me a tenner I'd end up playing at least a dozen games that season. I don't know if that was a motivational thing, but I ended up getting my money.

Getting as many games as I did so early on was more than I'd expected. When I made the first-team squad, Bolton already had an established and experienced duo at the back in the form of Mark Winstanley and Mark Came. I knew my chances would be limited to when one or the other was unavailable. As it turned out, those chances came earlier on than I'd been expecting. I played in the pre-season Lancashire Manx Cup in place of Mark Winstanley, where we beat Burnley 3–0: according to the local *Bolton Evening News,* 'Stubbs did well enough in place of Winstanley to confirm he had the qualities to be drafted in when necessary'.

A couple of weeks later, I made my league debut as Bolton lost 1–0 away at Bradford City: I came on for Mark Came once we were a goal down, with Phil Neal telling the press he felt 'let down by his central defenders . . . I could have pulled either of them off.' A couple of days later, Bolton were at home to Huddersfield for the first round, second leg of the Rumbelows Cup (as the League Cup was called then). Phil decided it was a good opportunity to give me a proper run out, and I found myself starting alongside Mark Winstanley.

It was my full senior debut, and it couldn't have started any better: only six minutes into the game, I found myself on the scoresheet. Our striker, Tony Philliskirk had crossed the ball in, only for the Huddersfield goalkeeper to spill it. I was in the right place, stuck my foot out and jabbed it into the net. It was a fantastic start. It also sealed the tie as a contest, as we were already 3–0 up from the first leg. We went on to win 2–1, I ended up being voted man of the match, and as the League Cup was sponsored by Rumbelows, I was presented with a 21-inch colour TV complete with Teletext and cheesy photo-opportunity in the local press ('Stubbs in the Frame').

I don't know how much Phil was intending to play me over the following weeks, but later on in that match Mark Winstanley was sent off for a professional foul. It was a harsh decision – this was right after the 1990 World Cup, and I think that referees were still getting their heads round the new rules about denying goals-coring opportunities. The upshot for me was that Mark was now facing a ban for three games as a result. The ban didn't come in straightaway, and Mark and I continued our partnership for the next match. That was also against Huddersfield, this time in the league, and wasn't such a success: we lost 4–0, having a player sent off after only half an hour. As Mark's ban came in, Phil paired me up with the club's other centre-half, Dean Crombie. We played together for two matches and suffered two further defeats.

It wasn't the start to the campaign that Bolton had been expect-ing. The club had finished sixth the previous season, losing to Notts County in the play-offs. Phil Brown had claimed at the start of the season in the press that 'nothing less than automatic promotion' would be sufficient. By the end of September, however, we'd only won two out of our first seven games. The club moved swiftly to rectify this, bringing in Sammy Lee to bolster the midfield and signing the central defender Mark Seagraves from Manchester City. Seagraves cost £100,000 and was clearly bought to go straight into the side. I was back down the pecking order, and would have to wait until later in the season for my chance to come again.

I didn't begrudge that at all. Being a central defender might not always be the most glamorous position in the side, but it's a crucial one, as more often than not you're matched up against the best players in the opposition team. So there's a lot of responsibil-ity on your shoulders when you're picked there. I was still a young player and finding my way: as with any rookie, you make mistakes and it takes a while for you to become consistent. With those early matches, the opportunities arose because of injuries and sendings-off. That meant I ended up playing alongside different players – it almost felt like a different player for every match. That's never good in terms of getting settled; it was only towards the end of that season that I had the chance for an extended run alongside Mark Seagraves.

Despite the chopping and changing of partnerships, I still learnt a lot from playing alongside these older, more experienced players, and training with them, too. Mark Winstanley, particularly, was very helpful right from the start. He was a tough defender, very hard and thickset but a lovely guy underneath. He was from down south, and had your classic west country 'Combine Harvester' type accent. He could have been quite off with me – I was a young guy in competition with him for a place in the team – but he was always helpful. Mark Came, by contrast, kept himself to himself: he wasn't much of a talker on the pitch, and once training or the match had finished, he'd be away. I don't know what he thought of me: even at eighteen I wasn't shy in telling people what I thought on the pitch. As far as I was concerned, I wasn't going to stand on ceremony; if I could see danger on the pitch, I'd let the others know.

There was a good group spirit at Bolton, even in those early games when things weren't going so well. The team socialised together, which I've always found to be important, and great for someone like me to get to know the other players. It was quite old school – we'd usually have the Wednesday off, so straight after training on a Tuesday, there'd be a move to head to the pub. If the team were playing Saturday, then everyone would meet up on the Sunday, too. I don't think that happens in quite the same way now: the culture has changed with the influx of foreign coaches and managers into the Premier League. But I still think the idea of meeting up and bonding is an important one, even if it is just for a meal and a couple of drinks. Certainly when I was at Celtic, that became an important part of pulling the team together.

Back at the start of the nineties, thoughts about drinking and dieting were some way off what has become the received wisdom of today. Diet was something that was pretty much left to the players to figure out for themselves. We'd get our weight checked at the start of the season and then again at Christmas time, and that would be about it. When Bruce Rioch became manager, he used to weigh us every few weeks and that felt quite a sea change.

Following the slow start to the 1990–91 season, things began to pick up. Mark Seagraves was a great addition to the team, and although Sammy Lee didn't play that many games, he was great to have around. I'd sometimes get a lift with him from Liverpool and he was a stickler for timekeeping. He absolutely hated it if you were running late – you could see it written all over his face. But he was a top, top player and gave the team a boost at just the right time.

Long term, it was the signing of Mark Seagraves that really helped the team. As I say, it restricted my appearances at first – I was back in the reserves for the middle part of the season – but as the club began to climb the table, we found ourselves forming a partnership. For the last fifteen games or so, we became the heart of the Bolton defence and worked well as a unit. It was nice to give the fans something to sing about, and equally not to have them on our backs. Burnden Park was a strange ground in some respects: it had the back of this supermarket at one end, and where once 60,000 people would cram in, now crowds of five or six thousand were more common. When crowds are smaller like that, you can hear more of what people were saying, and it didn't seem to take long for the crowd to turn. In one of my early matches, Bolton were playing Crewe Alexandra, and although we went on to win 3–2, we were two-down at half-time and got roundly booed off. One of the advantages of being a central defender is that you're not too close to the touchline and so escape some of the comments and criticisms: even so, when someone is shouting 'Come on Stubbs, pull your finger out!' it's difficult to ignore completely.

As the season went on, the team started to win and the attendances began to rise. After a shaky start, we ended up finishing fourth, just three points off the top; we missed out on automatic promotion on goal difference. We then beat Bury over two legs to set up a play-off decider against Tranmere at Wembley. That was an experience and a half, to finish your first season as a professional playing there. As a young lad growing up, playing at Wembley was one of those things you always dream about. I'd always been someone who'd enjoyed the whole of FA Cup final day, watching the television coverage from ten in the morning to enjoy all of the pre-match build up.

Tranmere had finished below us in the league, but we knew it was going to be a tough game. They weren't an easy team to play against: they had a lot of Scousers in the team and were very vocal on the pitch. They weren't a particularly dirty team, but certainly weren't averse to putting the foot in, and made it difficult for us to play our game. I think it was one of those games where neither team were out and out favourites, and that was reflected in the match itself. After ninety minutes the score was still 0–0. It was only into extra-time that the deadlock was broken, and to the dismay of the Bolton fans and players, it was Tranmere who scored it.

The play-offs can be cruel, particularly if you're the team that finished higher up the table. We might have had a better record than Tranmere over the season, but that counted for nothing once the ref had blown his whistle to start the game. It was a disappointing way to end the season – all the anticipation of playing at Wembley, all the noise and excitement of being there. Yet even though we had been beaten, it just made me all the more determined to come back and win there. The next time Bolton played in a play-off final at Wembley, I was able to make amends.

If my first season as a professional had been quite a ride, my second, in every way, was something of a disappointment. Having come so close to promotion, the following season we were nowhere near. We ended up finishing mid-table in thirteenth place, twelve points adrift of even the final play-off place. For whatever reason, it just didn't happen that season. I don't know if it was the disappointment of not having gone up, or whether it was the added expectation of being favourites for promotion. It was probably a bit of both to be honest: opposition teams saw us as something of a scalp and raised their game accordingly.

For me, too, the defensive partnership I'd built up with Mark Seagraves was broken up. Phil Neal paired him up with Mark Winstanley or Mark Came for most of the season, and when I did get a game, I found myself in the team as a defensive midfielder. I didn't mind that so much: I saw it as a bit of a short-term fix and was happy to help the team out. Looking back, it also helped me to play there, and gave me a better understanding of the game. I'd always been comfortable with the ball, and knew I could pass: playing in midfield, with more going on, I had to learn to be that bit quicker in my decision making.

At the end of the season, Phil resigned. He'd been at the club seven years and I think he felt he'd taken the club as far as he could. His replacement, Bruce Rioch, turned out to be one of the biggest influences in my career. He was a strong character, no doubt about that. He was a very proud, almost regimental man: his father, indeed several members of his family, had been in the army, and that drive and discipline rubbed off on him. As a player, Bruce had been known to be a tough, hard, no-nonsense sort of player: some people thought he was dirty, though he'd say himself he was always hard but fair. He immediately instilled some of that into how we played. Phil Neal had always wanted Bolton to play, and put an emphasis on getting the ball forward as quickly as possible. Bruce's teams still had that flair to attack, but he also wanted them to be very hard to beat.

Right from the off, he worked us hard defensively. He wanted the team to defend together, from the strikers backwards. We practised defensively as a unit, getting to know our positions and where we should be on the pitch. But Bruce still wanted us to go forwards. As well as being a hard player, he also had a fantastic left foot on him, as he'd show us in training. This was reflected in him encouraging me to go forwards and play the ball out from the back. I remember one day I made the mistake of trying to dribble the ball out of defence. He dragged me to one side, and I thought, 'Here we go, I'm for it now'. But rather than bollock me for making a mistake, his response was the opposite: 'If you stop doing what you just did because you made a mistake, then I'll kill you.' So I had this encouragement and support to play, which I really appreciated.

Bruce was fantastic with me, which wasn't true for all the players. He had a real nasty edge to him when he wanted to. He could cut through you with one look and if you got on the wrong side of him that was it: you were finished. He would be quite happy to leave you to rot. Bruce could be a right bastard when he wanted to be.

Bruce would always take part in the practice games on the training ground, and for anyone he thought was out of line or who said something out of turn, he would wait for his moment, and do them: a proper old school going over, taking the player out and lifting them up off the floor. If that sort of incident happened between two players, you'd expect some sort of confrontation. But if you're clobbered like that by your manager? Bruce would stand over them and say, 'What are you going to do about it?' The player involved knew there wasn't anything he could do. He was just going to have to sit there and take it.

I don't think he wanted to make the players scared of him, but he wanted them to know who was in charge: you're welcome to have a go, he was saying in effect, but be prepared for the consequences. I don't think players mind that. It's good to see a manager who is passionate. It would be the same in the dressing room: sometimes you want a bit of emotion from the manager to get you going. Bruce would bawl at us, believe me. When he lost it, he would properly let everything go. He'd throw things and kick things – anything in his path would get it.

Does that work as a motivation technique? To be honest, I'd say about 75 per cent of the time, it's a waste of the manager's breath. Once you've heard the manager lose his rag at half-time, it doesn't quite have the same impact the next time they do it. Now I'm on the other side, I can see that. I've torn into my players but have come away thinking, was that really for their benefit, or for mine? It is a very thin dividing line. I suspect it's as much for my own self-satisfaction and letting off steam as it is about getting your point across. It's good for the players to see you're passionate, but if you're unhappy at the performance, you're probably as effective speaking to them in a low, menacing tone.

That's the theory. When you're managing yourself, it's not always easy to keep calm and carry on. I've certainly gone in at half-time and if anything is in my way, I know it's going to get kicked. A couple of seasons ago, I was up in Scotland managing the Everton reserves against Clyde. We were playing their first team, but our young lads started really well, and we should have been a couple of goals up. Instead, they go down the wing, put the ball in and score. The young lad who was covering should have done better and I was so furious with him, I spun round and punched the dugout. Usually, they have a bit of padding on the top, in case you bang your head when getting in. Not this one. I punched straight through and, wallop!!, smacked my hand against the metal frame. I hit it really hard, but because I was fuming and the adrenaline was pumping, I didn't really feel it at first. But then, when I turned back to the pitch – Christ, it was sore. Within about twenty seconds it had started to swell. By the time the team were in for half-time, I had an ice pack strapped to my hand – I had broken it, and was lucky not to have it put into a cast. So yes, I learned the hard way that losing your temper as a coach can be self-defeating.

All of that, though, was only one side of Bruce as a manager. For me and the other younger players like Jason McAteer, Bruce was never anything less than brilliant: he was like a father figure, so much so that some of the other players joked that we were his sons. Bruce could see that he had some decent players on his hands, who could be coached through to the next level, and he took us under his wing.

It was brilliant to have that support. The way Bruce looked after me and Jason was something else I have tried to learn from and pick up on with my own coaching. I said how the other players joked that we were like his sons, and it's interesting to see the similarities between coaching young players and parenting. There's no doubt that having children of my own has been a big help in being a coach: just as you work out what makes your children tick, so you do with the players as well. I'm really aware, too, that with some of the young lads they'll be spending more time with me than they will their own parents. That's a lot of responsibility: we having a saying at Everton that not every young player that comes through our door is going to become a footballer, but we can ensure that they leave a better person than when they came in.

That's a challenge. The way the game is now is different to when I started out at Bolton. There can be a bit more arrogance and cockiness to the younger players. They'll say something back to a first-team player in a way I'd never have dreamed of: I was of a generation that wouldn't even enter the first-team dressing room without knocking first. The chores and tasks I used to do have gone as well: the PFA have got involved, and now the young players can't be made to clean the baths, sweep the stands and so on. The responsibility that a coach or a manager has for their young players hasn't changed. But the recourse we used to have at our fingertips to deal with them has.

Bruce worked wonders on the younger players at Bolton, but his man management skills didn't just work on us: he brought in a player called Tony Kelly who had been around the lower divisions but was a fantastic footballer. We nicknamed him Zico for what he could do with a ball. Tony was too good, really, to be playing at this level, but he liked his food and drink. With Bruce in charge, Tony knew that he'd be on the scales first thing Monday morning, and this petrified him. He'd go on a bender on Saturday night, and then go into a strict routine to make sure he wasn't overweight. Under Bruce, he kept his weight down and flourished as a result.

He was strict, Bruce, no doubt about that. He kept tabs on your weight and fined you if were over. He was one for punctuality, too, and would fine you if you turned up late. He'd clearly thought about everything – he had a whole regime he wanted his players to follow. Training was harder work than it had been under Phil Neal: the tempo was definitely quicker, and it was both more structured and more physical. Sometimes in training, you can do sessions where there aren't many tackles going in. For Bruce, the more contact there was, the better.

His interest in our weight was probably the first steps towards what we know today as sports science. Attention was paid to diet and nutrition and advice was given on what we should and shouldn't eat. Nothing particularly groundbreaking: stay away from McDonald's, burgers and things like that. If you are having sausages, grill them rather than fry them and the same with bacon. It's not rocket science to realise that as a professional footballer you can't have an unhealthy diet. But the advice on what we should eat, and how it could improve our performance, was really useful to hear.

Gym work was something else that was starting to be encouraged. Bolton didn't have a gym at the time, more of a room with some weights in, a bicycle and a bench press. So I'd go down to the gym near where I lived, because the facilities were better. I wasn't big on weights; I was more interested in developing my 'core' – sit ups and so on, and using that as your strength. Lifting weights was all very well and you get some big muscles to show off, but it doesn't actually make you what I'd call 'football strong'. Being football strong is all about using your core, it's about movement to your right or your left, rather than flexing your biceps. At the time, a lot of this you worked out for yourself. These days, I think it's far more set out for players – they have their routines and programmes in the gym to work to.

Bruce's hard work and leadership was to pay off handsomely: in his three seasons in charge, the club was promoted twice, reached the final of the League Cup and scalped several leading Premier League clubs in cup competitions along the way. In the 1992–93 season, Bolton finished second, with a points total thirty higher than the season before. The final match of the season was about as old fashioned a football match as you could get: Bolton Wanderers versus Preston North End. We knew we needed to win to secure the automatic spot and as the match went on and the score was goalless, word filtered onto the terraces that Port Vale, our rivals for second place, were winning – if the results stayed the same, they would have been pipped us for promotion. Then we got a penalty with about fifteen minutes to go, which John McGinlay scored. At the end of the game, the fans poured onto the pitch to celebrate – it was the first time Bolton had been back in the second tier of English football for over a decade.

Bruce's first season in charge brought success in the cup as well as the league. In the third round of the FA Cup, the club were drawn against Liverpool: the first match at Burnden Park finished 2–2, before Bolton beat Liverpool at Anfield in the replay. I didn't play in those matches – almost the only games that season I missed – but as you can imagine, seeing Liverpool lose, and to a lower league team, was always a good feeling.

The following season saw an FA Cup draw with even more personal interest to it: this time the third round draw saw us paired up with Everton. That was a weird experience, for sure. The first match was at Bolton, and all my friends and family wanted tickets. That caused a bit of a kerfuffle because I got them tickets for the main stand. As soon as Everton scored, they were all up out of their seats, celebrating and cheering – right in the middle of the Bolton section. It took a while for them to explain who they were, and for everything to calm down: at one point it looked like they were going to be thrown out!

The match ended up 1–1, and the replay was set up for Goodison. I was nervous about that for all sorts of reasons. I'd always dreamed of playing there, I'd just never imagined it would be against, rather than for, Everton. I knew the stadium well, of course, and exactly the sort of reception we were likely to get. I was also nervous, too, on a personal level. There were stories in the papers about me being linked with other clubs, and although I wasn't thinking about moving, I was aware that I was going to be watched.

My family were all excited because they were going to Goodison, but it was a bittersweet occasion for me. I was professional about it, however. Irrespective of my being an Everton fan, I played for Bolton and that was the team I was there for. There was no doubt about that from my performance: having beaten Liverpool in a cup replay the previous season, Bolton now did the double by knocking out Everton too. We won 3–2, and to get me even more stick from my Everton mates, I scored as well! I'd like to say I didn't celebrate, but as a central defender I didn't score that often, so I suspect I did.

My dad, despite being an Everton fan, was chuffed that we had won. He was like any other Kirkby man: he wanted his son to win, whichever team he was playing against. It was an emotional occasion for me, but a fantastic experience. The atmosphere was amazing, and the crowd were superb. I came away thinking that even if I never ended up playing for Everton, I could say that I'd gone to Goodison and come away on the winning team.

Our reward for victory was everything we could have hoped for: Arsenal at home. This was their vintage team, with their celebrated back four of Adams, Bould, Winterburn and Dixon, with Seaman behind them in goal. There was no better defence probably in European football: they were basically the unbreakables. For me as a defender, I was in awe of what they did, and also nervous about the strikers I was to be coming up against: Paul Merson and, in particular, Ian Wright.

Once again it was a tremendous game at Burnden Park, and once again we held our own. The game finished 2–2, and we found ourselves heading down to Highbury for the replay. I don't know how many people fancied us for that, but we came away with a famous 3–1 victory. To put three past that defence on their home ground was quite an achievement. The game had been 1–1 after ninety minutes, so to keep going and get those goals in extra-time said everything about the team that Bruce had created. We had endeavour, guts and energy, and kept going until the final whistle. When you've got all that, anything is possible.

A result like that doesn't just give you confidence as a team, it also gives you that as a player. It's exciting to pitch yourself against the best players and see whether or not you have it in you to step up and handle them. Ian Wright was a handful over those two games, no doubt about it. My God, the guy could talk. He didn't shut up the entire match, just jabbering away in my ear trying to wind me up and put me off. Not in a nasty, sledging way, but cracking jokes and giving me a running commentary on the game, all the time trying to break my concentration.

'Your guy there, he's shit, isn't he . . . oh, how about that . . . great ball there, nice bit of skill . . .' Before I knew it, he has pulled off my shoulder and was running into space, leaving me for dust! Then as soon as the move broke down, he'd be back there again, jabbering away. Ian was complimentary, too, and would praise you when you did something well: 'Tell you what pal, what a fantastic bit of skill that was.' At the end of the match, he came up to me and shook my hand and said, 'I tell you what, you were fantastic, tonight.' I really appreciated that.

The victories over Liverpool and Everton were great experiences, but it was the Arsenal victory that really put us on the map as a young team going places. To win at Highbury under the lights was a special feeling; to become only the second team to beat them in almost thirty cup matches made it more so. We might only have finished mid-table in our first season in Division One, but that result was our calling card for what was to come. Just as with the Everton and Liverpool matches, we hadn't fluked a 1–0 win but held our own at home and done the business away. That was the first time that people sat up and took notice of us

– myself, Jason McAteer and Alan Thompson as young, up and coming players, and quality talent like John McGinlay, Andy Walker, David Lee, Owen Coyle and Tony Kelly. We had the makings of a proper team and it was exciting to think just how far we could go.

# 5

## A Double Dose of Wembley

The second season Bolton were in Division One, it all just came together: the style with which the team were playing, and the young age of the squad, seemed to stretch back to the club's glory days. Nat Lofthouse was club president at the time, so that link was always there. He'd always be around and would speak to the players – a really lovely guy. It helped that Bolton were doing well, but everyone involved in the club were extremely friendly and there was a genuine family feel. It wasn't a huge staff: we probably had six to ten people that we were seeing on a daily basis – the secretary, the people in the ticket office, the groundsman, a couple on the commercial side. That was it – you tended to see the same faces every day, and that helped generate real spirit.

The same was true of the town. Bolton was one of those places where the football team played a large part in the town's local identity. As the goals went in, so the fans came back, and that spurred the team on more. There was a real buzz about the place: you'd go into the city centre and you could feel the effect that the club's success was having on people. The fact that the team was so young was definitely part of that: we might not have had the largest squad in the division, but we had energy and fresh legs. The young team helped the town feel young again, too.

This spirit and sense of togetherness spilled over onto the pitch. We had quality players, for sure, but more than that, the Bolton team were a *team*, in terms of how we played. One of the things I've learnt in football over the years is that as good as your best players are, the other players in the team are just as important. You might have a brilliant striker or midfielder, but they can't be everywhere on the pitch: it's the way the lesser players perform, and their will to win, that is crucial to a team's success. The 'water-carriers' might not be as famous, but every great side needs them. It is all too easy to forget sometimes that football is a team game, not an individual one.

It was that team spirit that carried us through the 1994–95 season, and to the remarkable success we had. The FA Cup results in the previous seasons against Liverpool, Everton and Arsenal had left us feeling we could compete at the highest level. This felt like our chance to see if we could get there. We might only have finished fourteenth the previous season, but Bruce encouraged us to believe that promotion to the Premier League was a real possibility.

Before we got to that, there was another cup run to savour. This time it was the League Cup rather than the FA Cup, and this time we were to make it all the way to Wembley: something that is always a huge achievement for a club from the lower tiers. We did it the hard way, beating first Ipswich and then Sheffield United with the help of an own goal, then claiming two Premier League scalps in the form of West Ham and Norwich. This set us up for a two-legged semi-final against Swindon. For once, we found ourselves in the position of being favourites – Swindon were struggling at the wrong end of the table, but the difference in our league position counted for nothing.

We played the first leg down in Wiltshire, where we lost 2–1. It could have been worse: I'd scored to keep us in the tie, and we were relieved to get back to Lancashire only a goal down. Back at Burnden Park, we felt it would be a different matter. Having got the away goal, we only needed to win 1–0 to go through. The atmosphere that night was incredible. There was a crowd of just under 20,000 people squeezed into the groaning old stadium, and it was exactly what you wanted it to be: noisy, hostile and intimidating to the away team. Swindon, though, weren't phased. Half-time came and went with the game still goalless: as hard as we tried, we couldn't find a way through. Then it all seemed to go wrong. Out of nowhere, Jan Fjortoft cropped up to score for Swindon after 53 minutes. They were 1–0 up on the night, 3–1 up on aggregate. Because they had the away goal in the bag, it meant we now needed three goals in just over half an hour to go through.

It was a real character test. To be that close to Wembley, and for the chance to be slipping away, it was hard not to let your head go down. You could tell from the crowd's reaction, too, exactly what they thought. And yet, somehow we came through. This was a team that never knew when it was beaten, and who would fight until the last. Bruce made a couple of substitutions, gave Jason McAteer more licence to roam in midfield and brought Mixu Paatelainen on off the bench. The changes turned out to be inspired stuff. Jason scored our first goal, putting away the rebound after Alan Thompson had hit the post; then Mixu walloped a shot in from 25 yards out. From looking dead and buried, we were now ahead on the night and all-square on aggregate. The crowd switched from restless to right behind us, willing us to go forward and win. The goal that got us to Wembley came just three minutes before the end, John McGinlay scoring our third after a free-kick had rebounded back to him.

Semi-finals can be a funny affair. They seldom make great games because neither team wants to lose so close to the final. There's definitely an element of it not mattering how you get through as long as you do, and that was certainly the case that night. But our victory was also down to our belief as a side – we had a bit of fire in our belly. If you look at our results in the league that season, we won a lot of games late on. It's a good habit for a team to get into – however the first sixty, seventy minutes of the game has gone, you always believe that you still have a chance.

My only previous Wembley experience had been the play-off final against Tranmere in my first season as a professional. This time it was the real deal: a cup final, a full house and a top drawer opponent. Liverpool were in their 'Spice Boys' pomp, and boasted the likes of Robbie Fowler, Jamie Redknapp and Steve McManaman in their ranks, alongside old hands such as John Barnes and Ian Rush. The atmosphere in Bolton leading up to the match was brilliant; the club took 25,000 fans down, which considering the average gate at this point was 10–15,000, was pretty impressive. It really felt like the whole town was behind us, and the team desperately wanted to do our best for them.

We went down a few days before the match and stayed in the Sopwell House Hotel near St Albans, a venue that many clubs use before a cup final. We didn't train at Wembley, if I remember rightly: the first time we went down to the stadium was on the day itself. Arriving there about an hour and forty-five before the kick-off, we walked out onto the pitch in our suits and had a good look round. Some of the older players in the team like John McGinlay and Mark Seagraves tried to tell the younger lads to soak up the atmosphere. Take it all in, they told us, because it will go by so quickly.

The fact that it was Liverpool we were up against made the day extra special for me. I'd grown up at the same time as some of their players – Steve McManaman, for example, I'd been playing matches against since I was a young boy. Now here we were, facing each other again at Wembley. Stevie was someone who'd always been a talent right from the early days. He had great balance, was brilliant at moving the ball left to right and a fantastic dribbler. When he was on song, he could go past players at will. Even when he was twelve, he was someone you watched and thought: he'll be a professional one day.

Stevie wasn't even the best of our generation, curiously enough: there was another lad, Danny, who was better than all of us. He went to Liverpool, I think, but there were a few incidents and he got released. Strange how that happens sometimes: there was another player from Kirkby called John O'Leary who Bobby Charlton once famously described as the best player he'd ever seen. He had all the clubs after him, but for whatever reason decided not to make a go of it.

There was a bit of an edge to the match itself, especially among the Scousers. There was all the typical banter – 'you're shit', 'you're crap', 'God, you're having a nightmare' – and a little kick here or there when the ball is coming in, leaving your elbows out and your foot in. Remember, we'd beaten them in the FA Cup a couple of seasons before, and they were desperate for that not to happen again.

I enjoyed playing at Wembley. I think I've always been a big game player. That's not true of every footballer and was the same at Celtic: you could look around the pitch and see the body language of your team-mates, who's shoulders were out and who's were in. I loved everything about that experience, everything except for the result. We played well, there's no doubt about that, and in the first half created the best chances. But somehow they got the goal – it was McManaman (who else?) who cut in, gave me the slip and scored. After the break, we were comfortably on top, and had the bulk of possession. Once again though, it was Stevie who did for us – another mazy run against the run of play and we were 2–0 down. We pulled one back through Alan Thompson, and gave it a real go for the last twenty minutes. But it wasn't quite enough and Liverpool held on.

Were Liverpool the better team? Not on the day. Did they have better quality? Bolton had quality in areas, but we didn't have it in depth like they had. They had individuals we couldn't deal with: Stevie was excellent and won the game for them with two moments of brilliance. I was devastated after the match, absolutely. I was gutted because I knew we had come close, and felt that we had had a real chance of winning. The Liverpool players knew that too: that we deserved more and that they'd been given a tough game. But the best team on the day doesn't always end up on top. It was a fantastic occasion, and one that will always live with me. It was just a shame that we lost, and lost to Liverpool as well.

As it turned out, this wasn't going to be our last visit to Wembley that season. It would have been easy for Bolton to have suffered a post-final lull, but with automatic promotion a real possibility, we had to push on. We recorded back-to-back wins the week after the final, and were in a great position for a top-two finish. But then came a disappointing end to the season – we won only one of our last seven fixtures, and we ended up finishing third. It was play-off time again, with Bolton up against Wolves, and Reading against Tranmere in the other match.

Just as in the League Cup semi-final against Swindon, we lost the first leg away from home, 2–1. Our regular goalkeeper, Keith Branagan, was unavailable, but we had the best possible replacement drafted in: the legendary Peter Shilton. We were grateful he was there, especially when we had Neil McDonald sent off and had to play out the game with ten men. Already 2–1 up, Wolves laid siege to our goal, and it was only thanks to a number of great saves from Peter that they didn't take the tie away from us. The return leg, as against Swindon, was a tense affair. This time, however, John McGinlay got a goal before half-time to settle the nerves and level the scores on aggregate. It wasn't until well into extra-time, however, that John scored again – the first time we'd been in front over the two legs. That was the way it stayed, and we were back to Wembley again, for a play-off final against Reading: a match that no one who saw it would ever forget.

It was the second time we'd play under the twin towers in two months, but any sense that our experience of having already played there might give us an advantage was quickly dispelled. Once again we found ourselves 2–0 down, but this time after only twelve minutes. It was a horror start and looked like it was going to get even worse. Ten minutes before half-time, Jason McAteer brought down Michael Gilkes and the referee pointed to the spot. If we'd gone 3–0 down before half-time, even with our resilience, that probably would have been it. But Keith Branagan, back in goal, was a hero: he guessed right and saved the penalty. That felt like a big moment – from that point on, getting back into the game didn't feel insurmountable.

Once again, Bruce did his job at half-time. He brought on Fabian de Freitas, which was a bit of a gamble: Fabian was tall, gangly and fast, but also a bit of an enigma. Sometimes he was great, at other times all over the place: you never knew quite what you were going to get. Bruce got the call right, and Wembley turned out to be one of Fabian's days. You could see immediately that the Reading defence didn't like his pace, and before long we'd pulled one back, Owen Coyle heading home. Then just before the end of normal time, Fabian scored the equaliser.

The atmosphere in Wembley by this point had completely turned around. The momentum on the pitch was with us; in the stands, it was our fans who were making all the noise. The game went into extra-time, and you just felt there was only going to be one winner. Mixu Paateleinen put us ahead after being fed by John McGinlay, and then Fabian scored again with three minutes of extra-time remaining. Reading pulled one back to make it 4–3 with a minute to go, but it was too late. We'd won the match, and promotion to the Premier League.

By this point in my Bolton career, I was club captain, which meant I took the players up the famous steps to get the trophy. It had raised a few eyebrows when Bruce had originally passed me the armband. But it made sense: I'd always been a leader on the pitch and being captain was an extension of that. I think Bruce also wanted to emphasise that his Bolton side was a youthful team with the potential to go places.

Every other time I'd been to Wembley, either as a player or as an Everton fan, had ended up in defeat, so it was a great feeling this time. I knew in my gut we were going to do it, that it was going to be our day. It still lingers long in the memory, that afternoon. People who were there still talk about it, say how it was one of the best atmospheres they'd ever experienced at a football match. It was one of those special Wembley days. I liked what they'd done with the new stadium – I went there with Everton as part of the coaching staff, and the way the noise holds is wonderful – but there was something iconic about winning under those twin towers. It was what I dreamt about growing up, so to captain the winning team for such a memorable match was very special.

It was party time. We returned to the hotel – all the wives and families and friends came back. There was food and drinks laid on, and we celebrated well into the night. The play-off match for the Premier League has been called the most expensive match in football, with its prize of tens of millions of pounds for the winner.

As a player, you don't think about the money aspect so much. It's more about getting into the top division and having the chance to play against the best teams. We'd had a flavour of that in the various league and FA Cup matches over the previous two seasons. Now it was going to be a chance to prove ourselves, week in, week out, against the top players.

I certainly felt I was ready for the challenge. As Bolton had been doing well that season, there had started to be rumours here and there about how this club or that team were having a look at me. All of which had been boosted by the fact that at the end of the previous season, I'd been picked to play for the England 'B' team, in a match against Northern Ireland. It was a complete surprise when the call came through. They rang the club, and Bruce called me into the office to tell me the news. Considering I wasn't even playing in the Premier League at this point, and I was just twenty-two, it felt a huge achievement, and nice to know that people were out there watching me.

The match was played at Hillsborough, Sheffield Wednesday's ground. It was great to walk in and see all the kit laid out – your England kit. You got your cap, too. I found it the other day, funnily enough, going through the loft looking for something. I've never been one for nostalgia and medals: my reward was always playing the games themselves. There were some great players in the team – this was right at the start of the Terry Venables era, and his putting together a side that would get to the semi-finals of Euro 96. There were some good players in the team that night – Steve Bould was captain, and also on the pitch were Paul Merson, Rob Lee and a young Chris Sutton. I came on as a sub for Chris Bart-Williams, and it was a nice moment, for sure, to go out and represent your country. It was quite slow, that was what I really remember of the match: it was all about possession, rather than the pace I was used to playing at. England were already

81

winning 3–2 when I came on, and scored again at the end to put the match beyond doubt.

They're funny things, 'B' internationals, and they don't really have them any more. It would have been nice to have gone on and got a full cap, but for whatever reason it never quite happened. I was always quite realistic about my chances, rather than getting carried away at having been picked. There were some fantastic defenders around at the time – the likes of Tony Adams and Gareth Southgate, for example – so I knew my chances were always going to be limited. When I signed for Celtic, I knew that would most likely take me off the radar. Did I regret that? Not one bit. I was a club man, was all about club football, so when the phone calls didn't come, it was never something that bothered me. I'm not saying it wouldn't have been nice, but it was never something that kept me awake at night.

The contrast between the 1994–95 season when we got promotion and the 1995–96 season in the Premier League couldn't have been starker. As so often is the case, the seeds for relegation were sown over the summer, before a ball had been kicked. For all the euphoria of beating Reading at Wembley, we knew as players that the squad wasn't going to be good enough to survive. I had a lot of respect for the players who were there and had taken us up, but I knew we needed more quality if we were going to hold our own in the top division.

That called for investment. Middlesbrough, who were the other team to be promoted that season, were quick to get the chequebook out: this was the era of chairman Steve Gibson and Bryan Robson as manager, and they took the opportunity to improve their team. As club captain, I spoke with the chairman. I told him and the manager that we needed to get more quality players in, but for whatever reason they decided not to.

I felt it was a missed opportunity and showed a lack of ambition by the club.

Out of Bolton's promotions, it was the jump between Division One, as it was then, and the Premier League that was the biggest. That was the gulf in class that needed dealing with. That divide, I think, was wider than it is now. I don't think the Premier League is as strong now as it was back then: the Manchester United and Arsenal sides were extremely strong in the mid-nineties and from there downwards, there was depth throughout the division. I think it was harder then for a team to come up and stay up than it is now. Without sounding brutal about it, that required money.

What also didn't help matters was the fact that shortly after Bolton were promoted, Bruce Rioch left to go and manage Arsenal. There had been rumours that he might leave, but even so, it was still a bit of a shock when the news came out. If I remember rightly, he addressed us as a team, told us that he'd had this opportunity and had decided to go. We were disappointed, of course, but no one begrudged him the chance. We knew we'd had a good manager and that the Arsenal job was a difficult one to turn down. If the decision was mine to make as a player, I knew I would have done exactly the same. Even so, it meant the players all left for our summer holidays a bit deflated. It seemed an incredibly short time from the heady excitement of Wembley to uncertainty as to how things were going to unfold.

For me personally, I was massively disappointed to see Bruce go. He had been a huge influence on my career and had really supported me, allowing me to play football as well as just defending. On top of which, Bruce had always been good to me in terms of contracts: I must have had four or five new ones while he was in charge. He'd have me in his office the whole time, would ask me how things were, tell me I was doing great, and give me another one to sign.

One time he had called me in and told me, 'Listen Alan, you've got to get yourself an advisor, an agent or someone to look after you.' I was still relatively young and didn't really know much about this side of the game. Bruce suggested that his brothers looked after me: Neil and Ian Rioch worked together as agents, with Ian the senior one, but Neil was the guy who really ran the company. I think Bruce had suggested them with the best of intentions: he wanted me to have someone professional to help me, but in retrospect, I should have gone with someone more impartial and also more qualified. When I signed for Celtic, there was an issue because the brothers weren't properly licensed, and FIFA stepped in and issued a forty grand fine. I didn't have a clue what was going on – as far as I was aware they were licensed. That was an eye-opener for me.

Bruce, it turned out, wasn't the only key component of the Bolton setup to leave. Right at the start of the new season, a call came in from Blackburn Rovers. Rovers at the time were the Premier League champions, with Kenny Dalglish's team pipping Manchester United to the title. Blackburn were interested in signing both myself and Jason McAteer, and offered £9 million for the pair of us in a joint deal. It was an all or nothing offer: Blackburn stipulated that no one else was allowed to talk to us, and that the deal was for both of us, or neither.

It was a lot of money for the mid-nineties. When Blackburn made a formal bid and asked to speak to Jason and me, Bolton accepted. We met up at the Thistle Haydock Hotel, just off the M6. Blackburn officials had booked a room and we went in and met Kenny Dalglish. Kenny was moving up to be Director of Football, with his assistant Ray Harford taking over the running of the team. Kenny's a legend, of course, and we were both impressed: Jason in particular, as a boyhood Liverpool fan, was bowled over. To be playing for the league champions alongside the likes of Alan Shearer and Chris Sutton was a tantalising thought. The agents settled down to do the negotiations and everything progressed smoothly.

Just as it seemed as though we were about to sign, Liverpool came in and made an offer of £4.5 million for Jason. Despite the exclusivity arrangement with Blackburn, Bolton decided to tell Jason and give him permission to speak to them. It was a tricky situation – Liverpool was Jason's team, but his signing would mean the Blackburn deal was off. He rang me up before he signed and we discussed it.

'They're my team, Alan,' he explained. 'I'm really sorry, but I can't turn down this opportunity.'

I understood. If it had been the other way round, with Everton coming in for me, I would have been exactly the same. I didn't have a problem with Jason doing that at all. If I was disappointed with anyone, it was Bolton. As soon as Blackburn found out about the Liverpool offer, they pulled the plug on the deal. I was left stranded and wondering what was going on. I hadn't asked for a transfer, but it's difficult to go through that sort of situation and not find it unsettling. With Bruce gone, and now Jason too, the Bolton dressing room felt a different place. That was symptomatic of the club's attitude to promotion – not only did the board not invest, we found ourselves entering the Premier League with the ranks depleted.

The new management team at Bolton was Colin Todd and Roy McFarland. They knew each other well and had an understanding back from their playing days together. They were a decent managerial unit: Roy was probably the better coach, with Toddy a quieter, 'take a step back' sort of person. He wasn't really a shouter, more of a talker and thinker. Together, they worked well and I can't say what happened to Bolton that season was down to them:

it was more about the fact that the club hadn't invested. They did what they could with the resources available.

The main difference I found about the Premier League, compared to playing in the lower divisions, was the speed of thought needed, and how little time you had to think and work out what was going on. As a defender, I was playing against players who played off your shoulder: the likes of an Andy Cole or an Alan Shearer. The problem was that I couldn't see both the player and the ball at the same time: if I was watching the ball, I couldn't see what the player was doing. I couldn't see that precise moment when they were peeling off and making space for themselves. People often talk about the pace of the Premier League, but it's the speed at which you have to think, and take everything in, that sets it apart.

For a defender, it's all about concentration. In the Championship or the lower leagues, you could make four or five mistakes in a game and get away with most of them. In League One or League Two, you might well get away with them all; in the Championship, you might get punished for one of those slip-ups. Step into the Premier League and those four or five mistakes could equal four or five goals. It's a vicious circle: once you find yourself at the wrong end of the table as Bolton did, then you are under more pressure; the more pressure you're under, the smaller the margin for error.

I don't think anyone was under any illusions about the club's chances during that season: seventeenth place was the target, right from the start of the season. When you have got that thought in your mind, it is never going to get any better than that. And it didn't. It was a shame; the fans were up for it, and so were the players. With a bit more optimism, I think we could have finished higher. As it was, the players quickly found their level: while some of the team could cut it, there were others who found it hard going. We were a young team, with very little Premier League experience, and it didn't take long for this to show. By the time this realisation had sunk in, Bolton were already doing badly and it was too late. The board just accepted it, effectively saying, okay, we'll take the money, go back down and rebuild our way up. That's what happened – Bolton became a 'yo-yo' club for a few years.

Nobody likes losing football matches, least of all me. What felt frustrating was that we'd put in all this hard work to get ourselves promoted and now, here we were, letting the opportunity pass us by. Rather than giving it our best shot, we let things drift away from us, going down with a whimper, rather than a bang. It's hard to play in that sort of atmosphere. We'd gone from a successful season, where we were used to winning, to one where we won two matches in five months: we beat Blackburn 2–1, where I scored the winning goal, and defeated Bruce Rioch's Arsenal, but that was it until the new year. Week in week out, those sort of results were difficult to take. It's a horrible place to be: we knew as a team we weren't good enough, but the decision had been made that nothing was going to be done to change it.

As a player, and also as a manager, that leaves you feeling exposed. Hard work will only ever get you so far. And we did work hard: we never gave up and there was only the odd match, against Manchester United (0–3) and Liverpool (2–5), that we were completely out of it. But for all the effort you put in, if the other team also works hard, and have quality on top of that, what chance do you have? Colin and Roy knew that: they gave us the occasional bollocking, but after a while thought 'we can't keep having a go at these players because it's not their fault'.

By about Christmas, the attitude changed. Everyone accepted that we weren't going to stay up, and the bollockings were replaced with, 'Listen lads, just go out there and do your best.'

Roy left, leaving Toddy in sole charge, and the ethos became, 'Let's just try and get through this season'. Pick up a few points, win a few games. Do things properly. And to be fair, that's what we did – in the second half of the season, we won half a dozen games. Whether that was because the pressure was off, or because we'd acclimatised a bit, I'm not sure. But it confirmed to me just what an unforgiving place the Premier League is. If you don't hit the ground running from the start, then you're always going to be in trouble.

I learnt a lot from the experience. As both a player and also in terms of thinking about coaching, it was all good stuff to bank. It didn't feel like it at the time, but it undoubtedly helped me, testing myself against so many fantastic players. It helped me, too, in terms of coping with defeat and dealing with bad runs. It's useful as a coach to have gone through that, to see what works in motivating players. It's useful, too, to experience what happens when you don't have the support, and what you need in terms of backup to be successful.

Bolton ended up finishing bottom, getting relegated with Queens Park Rangers and Manchester City. Immediately, the talk turned to getting Bolton back up. That's where things got a little strained. My relationship with Toddy had always been good, but it was clear that he expected me to stay and help the team get promoted. I was in a different place: I wanted to play in the Premier League and felt that was where I belonged. By this point, I'd been at Bolton for eight years, so didn't feel disloyal in thinking that.

Toddy, though, was not happy about the thought of me leaving. He started being a bit sharp with me around the training ground, snapping at me to get on with it, and that sort of thing. I knew what he was trying to do – he wanted to keep the team together and keep hold of his best players – but I didn't feel he was appreciating it from my point of view. I went to see the chairman Phil Garside, who by contrast couldn't have been nicer. He was lovely with me and listened to what I had to say.

'Stay one more season,' he asked me. 'If we don't go back up, then I will let you go.'

Then Celtic offered to make me their record signing.

# 6

## Welcome to Glasgow

Moving to Celtic was a big decision, both professionally and also personally. Mandy and I were married by this point and expecting our first child: she was heavily pregnant when the offer came in. It's funny how in life things often happen at once. All in all, it was a big deal moving away from Liverpool and our families. Mandy, though, has always been very supportive of me and my football. She was right behind me all the way, and never made things awkward for me about going.

I'll always be grateful to Mandy for that. Leaving Liverpool was difficult for us both, but probably more so for Mandy. We had been brought up in an area which was very family orientated, and where we had our parents, our siblings and our friends. To start again, especially when you're just having a baby, is not an easy thing to do. For me, my routine was set: I was up, off for training, and would be seeing and socialising with my new team-mates. Mandy didn't have that: she had a new place to live, new friends to make and a new baby to look after. At least her mum came up after the birth, which was a great help in those first few weeks.

I think we both found that transition harder than we were expecting. I missed my home comforts. I missed going out with and seeing our parents. I missed my old mates coming round for a cup of tea, or popping over to theirs; I missed going out for a drink with them on a Saturday night. What Mandy and I found in those early months was that whenever we had a chance, we would go back down to Liverpool. Wednesday would usually be my day off, so we'd head back down on Tuesday after training and return to Glasgow Thursday morning. Which was great in terms of seeing people, but less so in terms of settling in.

I had a lot on my mind. I was flattered that Celtic had paid so much money for me, but could also feel the £4.5 million price tag weighing heavily on my shoulders. To say I felt a lot of expectation was putting it mildly. The Gaffer, Tommy Burns, had said that he wanted the team shaped around me. Celtic had got this reputation at the time for having a slightly leaky defence, which my signing was there to stop. Because of the size of the club, and because it can feel sometimes like *everyone* in Glasgow, Scotland even, are either Celtic or Rangers, the pressure to pay back that faith is huge. The result was that on the pitch, as well as off it, it took a little while to settle.

The Celtic team were brilliant. Here I was, this guy coming up from England with a big price tag around my neck. It would have been the easiest thing in the world for them to try and take me down a peg or two, but they couldn't have been more welcoming. Even John Hughes – 'Yogi', as we called him – was friendly, despite the fact that it quickly became apparent he was the one earmarked to make way for me. There was a bit of banter about that, but it was all good-humoured, never with any malice.

There was a bit of joshing about my nationality, too. I was the only English guy there: fourteen of that original squad were Scottish, then there was me, and a handful of foreign players. The spirit in the squad was good; it was never cliquey or anything like that. And there were some right characters there. The only quiet one really was Jorge Cadete, the club's Portuguese striker. Jorge somehow seemed to get away with never having to train: whenever he could, he'd find a reason to get a massage. He was always on that masseuse table! No one minded, because he'd bang the goals in, so we'd leave him to it.

Up front with Jorge at the time was Paolo di Canio. He was quite someone to have around. Paolo is the hardest training foreign player I have ever come across. He was a fantastic footballer anyway, but his attitude to hard work and training was immense. He'd spit his dummy out, for sure. There were plenty of occasions where he would boot balls away because he was not happy with a decision, but I never minded it. He was the same as me in that he had this passion and desire to win.

Paolo also liked to look good. The guy was *always* in front of the mirror! He was always well turned out, had that bit of Italian style to him. But he'd spend so much time in front of the mirror, it was almost as if he was having a relationship with it: after training, no-one else could get anyway near it. He would spend ten minutes looking at himself, preening himself, gelling his hair back and shaving his chest.

'Bella Figa!' he'd say, admiring himself. 'My mother gave birth to a beautiful baby'.

'Get off the fucking mirror, Paolo,' we'd reply. 'Give someone else a chance, yeah?'

When he first joined Celtic, Paolo had been disappointed to discover that there were no bathrobes waiting for him to put on after he'd had a shower.

'But that's what we had at Milan,' he explained, which had been his previous club.

'Welcome to Glasgow', was the response.

We had some great players in that team. Pierre van Hooijdonk was another quality player. His English was good and he mingled with the lads. He wasn't afraid to express his thoughts; early on in that first season, Tommy left him out of a game and he told him to fuck off. He had quite a few run-ins like that. Pierre thought that he was the best player at the club, he thought he should always play and that he should be on the most money. When he suspected others were earning more than him, he wasn't happy at all. But that was all with the management: with the other players, he was great.

There was Malky Mackay, who'd come up via the unconventional route of working as a bank clerk while playing part time early in his career. He was a smart, clever guy, and I got on really well with him; his subsequent success as a manager doesn't surprise me at all. We had Peter Grant, who was nicknamed 'Peter the Pointer', because that's what he used to do all the time on the pitch; point and moan at the other players because he was so desperate to win. Andreas Thom was our flair player – fantastic ability, with the biggest legs you'd ever seen. Then there were the established Scottish internationals like Tosh McKinlay and Tommy Boyd, and up and coming players such as Jackie McNamara and Phil O'Donnell.

It was a fine squad and a really nice bunch of players. A few of us started going out after training on a Tuesday, and before long everyone wanted to come along. It quickly became a fixture and was great both in terms of me getting to know the other lads, and also in building team spirit. We'd meet at about four o'clock in the Italian Centre in Glasgow and have ourselves a late lunch. Paolo was completely in his element, chatting away to the staff who all loved him, and telling us what we should be eating. Before you knew it, it was seven o'clock; some of the lads would peel off home and the rest of us would stay out and go for a drink. It quickly became a weekly ritual and did wonders in creating a sense of togetherness.

We had a fantastic guy, too, in Tommy Burns, as our manager. He was still in that transition stage between being a player and a manager and was easily good enough to join in with our training. To be honest, I think he was still getting to grips with being a manager: he was a fan, too, and was so passionate about the club he'd sometimes get caught up in all that and would sometimes manage as a fan rather than as a manager. I sometimes think that the word 'class' is used too much, but in Tommy's case, the guy was pure class. I loved the guy, and everything that he stood for: his mannerisms, his sense of humour, his affection for both the players and the Celtic staff. He had an absolute aura about him and the players would do anything he asked of us.

Tommy's class showed through with how he dealt with Mandy and I settling in. We bought a house in Newton Mearns, which is a lovely area just outside Glasgow on the way to Ayrshire, and we probably settled into the house better than we did in Scotland in general, really. Having had our first child, Heather, Mandy became pregnant again, but sadly had a miscarriage. In fact, she had two miscarriages in our first year up there, which wasn't easy to deal with. That led to Mandy getting really homesick, and wanting to move closer to Liverpool. All of which had an effect on me: how could it not?

I went to see Tommy Burns and spoke to him about it.

'It's been a difficult start,' I explained. 'Mandy is finding it hard to settle and wants to get back home.'

Tommy was brilliant about it. He heard everything I said and wanted to help.

'Listen,' he said. 'Can we see whether we can work it out?'

'Sure,' I replied. 'But it is going to be difficult'.

In the meantime, I had changed agents: I had left the Rioch brothers after the incident with the licensing and had signed up with Paul Stretford. Paul knew the situation, too, and came up with a way out.

'If it doesn't work out at Celtic,' he told me, 'I know that Aston Villa are keen to sign you. I have had negotiations with them, and they are really interested in you playing for them.'

It turned out that Aston Villa had put an offer in to Celtic for £5 million. Celtic turned this down; Villa then offered £5.5 million and the club turned that down, too. They came back again and made a final offer of £6 million: Stretford, meanwhile, was keen to agree personal terms with them on the basis that the offer was going to be accepted. But the Celtic chairman, Fergus McCann, turned the offer down: he told Villa I had a valuation on the books of £6.5 million and Villa decided not to stretch that far. If the deal had been struck, I would probably have gone because of Mandy and wanting to get her closer to home. But it didn't go through and thankfully, it didn't leak out either. If the negotiations had come out at the time, that would certainly have made life more difficult.

Meantime, the club were brilliant with Mandy. Tommy started sending round his wife, Rosemary, to see Mandy. She would take her out to the shops, take her to coffee to meet people and show her Glasgow. The club said, too, that they wanted Mandy's mum to come up more and they helped to do that. From that point on, the situation began to improve. Mandy managed to meet a few people, make friends in the area and everything seemed to progress. That helped me enormously: knowing Mandy was settled made me relax too, and meant that I could concentrate on my performances on the pitch.

The first match I played at Celtic Park was a pre-season friendly against Arsenal. It had to be Arsenal, somehow, with Bruce Rioch as manager and bringing the team he tried to get me to join. It was strange seeing him there and we had a good chat about it all. He apologised for what happened, said that he was really sorry that it hadn't gone through.

'I wish you were in my team, rather than Celtic's,' he said ruefully, and wished me all the best for the future.

And what a future it was. Celtic Park is undoubtedly one of football's special venues. It was still in the middle of redevelopment when I started, with the Jock Stein stand opening in 1998 to create a capacity of just over 60,000. But even without this being completed, the place was still an extraordinary venue to play football in. That's partly because of the amazing support that Celtic has, and the passion they bring in getting behind their team. But it's also to do with the structure of the stadium: the way it holds the noise in, rather than letting it escape naturally. I had played in some big games in my career, had been to Wembley on a number of occasions, but Celtic Park took things to a new level. It was mind tingling: you walked out and could literally not hear yourself think.

I had to get used to that. In my first matches playing there, I remember shouting across to my team-mates – 'Hey, Andre! Boydy, Boydy, watch your man!' – and getting nothing back. I couldn't work out if they were blanking me, or if their mind was wandering off. Then I worked out that they couldn't hear what I was saying. It was the same the other way round – people yelling 'Stubbsy!' and me not responding back. Basically, unless the other player was within fifteen yards of you, you could forget it.

That was something I had to get used to. There'd be a bit of Chinese whispers going on from the dugout, with the manager telling someone on the touchline what he wanted, and the command would get passed across the field. When play stopped for a free-kick or someone getting treatment, those moments would be vital in getting information across. Communication was possible, but what I quickly learned about playing in such an atmosphere was that it was a lot about trust: you had to have complete faith in your team-mates that they knew what they were doing. It was also about preparation. We'd practise a lot of situations in training, so when they came up in a match, we'd know exactly what to do.

The atmosphere was part and parcel of being a Celtic player. If you wanted to succeed at the club, you had to be able to deal with that, and the pressure of playing with such support and expectation. I relished it, but quickly realised that it wasn't for everyone. There were some players who came to Celtic who simply couldn't deal with it. It wasn't that they were bad players, it was because they struggled to perform under the weight of all that. Signing for a big club is one thing; playing well for them is quite another.

We beat Arsenal 2–1 in that friendly, which was a great way to start. I couldn't wait for the season proper to begin, and didn't have long to wait for my competitive debut. We were away at Aberdeen and the contrast with that first start for Bolton couldn't have been greater. Then, I'd scored a goal after six minutes and ended up man of the match. Here, I was in the headlines again, but this time for all the wrong reasons.

Aberdeen had a pair of no-nonsense strikers up front in the form of Duncan Shearer and Dean Windass to deal with. They were a handful, but for most of the match I'd had them under control. Celtic were winning thanks to a first half goal from van Hooijdonk, but with about fifteen minutes to go, Dean slipped the ball through and it looked like Duncan might be away. I didn't hesitate and went for the ball. I still swear I got some of the ball with my boot, I definitely made contact, but because Duncan was sprinting through, I caught him in the process. I upset his momentum and he went down. From behind, which was where the referee was, you couldn't see I'd got the ball, just the striker going down in a heap in the penalty area. To make matters worse, I was the last defender: a potential red card offence.

The referee that day was Hugh Dallas. He reached for his pocket, sent me off and awarded Aberdeen a penalty. I was mortified. I protested my innocence, tried to explain that I'd got something on the ball, but it was to no avail. I had to leave the pitch. The Aberdeen fans, as you can imagine, absolutely loved it: here was Celtic's record signing, sent off on his debut. It was a long walk back to the dressing room and I sat there alone, head in my hands as I heard the roar that meant Aberdeen had equalised. Then, as Aberdeen pressed home their numerical advantage, I heard another roar as they made it 2–1. Andy Thom pulled one back for Celtic at the death to salvage a point, but it didn't make me feel much better. I didn't need to read the papers the next day: I knew exactly what the headline writers would say.

What I learnt the hard way that afternoon was how refereeing was going to be an issue throughout my time in Scotland. The reason it was an issue was because of the dominance of Celtic and Rangers in Scottish football.

Hugh Dallas was one of the top referees in the country, but from where I was standing on the pitch I felt he never needed much of an excuse to red card a Celtic player. That was part of a general Rangers–Celtic tension in refereeing that we had to deal with. In the opening three or four months of my first season in Scotland, Celtic had eight players sent off; Rangers, by contrast, hadn't had a player sent off for about two years. It was always denied, but it was a long-standing grievance at the club: as well as having to play your opponents on the pitch, there was a refereeing organisation that appeared more Rangers friendly. It wasn't cheating, I should be clear on that – but if there was a decision that could go one way or another, you just knew it would go against Celtic.

In England, there are quite clear rules about how referees aren't allowed to officiate in matches that involve the teams they support. So for example, Chris Foy is an Everton fan, and so he is never picked to referee the Blues; Mark Clattenburg is a Newcastle fan and so he doesn't officiate when they are playing. In Scotland, such was the dominance of Rangers and Celtic, it was more difficult to maintain such neutrality: if you took out all the Celtic and Rangers fans from the pool of potential referees, there wouldn't be many officials left. Add in the fact that each club has its associations with Catholicism and Protestantism, and it's easy to see how suspicions of bias can arise. In the January Old Firm game that season, we were losing 2–1, when we broke away and Jorge Cadete scored an equaliser. He was clearly onside, yet the linesman raised his flag and the goal was disallowed. I couldn't help asking myself whether the linesman was a Rangers fan. In such circumstances, it's difficult not to feel aggrieved.

I quickly learnt that in Scottish Football, everything was about Rangers and Celtic. Rangers, at this point, seemed to have all the cards stacked in their favour. This was a time when Rangers were the more successful side – they had won the title for a number of successive seasons – and they had some fantastic players like Brian Laudrup, Mark Hateley, Ally McCoist, Trevor Steven, . . . the list went on and on. They always seemed to have more money than us, the reasons for which would become clear years later.

Above all, they had Paul Gascoigne. Gazza was the outstanding player, both in terms of his footballing genius, and also in terms of the controversy that accompanied him. He was always on the edge, and as an opponent you were never quite sure what he was going to do next. He could show you up with a bit of skill on the pitch, or he could wind you up something rotten. There weren't many players who would happily shove a finger or their tongue in your ear, feel your arse, anything to get a response out of you. You'd turn round to say something and he'd have a big smile on his face. That was Gazza all over. It was unpredictable but never malicious.

I was unlucky that I had to play against Gazza in Scotland and then lucky that I got to play with him later on in my career at Everton. I got to know him pretty well – I'd see him for a drink up in Scotland, and when I first moved back down to Liverpool, spent some time staying in the same hotel as him. There are so many stories about Gazza, it's difficult to know where to start. There was the time that David Ginola signed for Everton, and at his first training session, Gazza came out wearing a long Ginola-style wig. He refused to take it off, and played the whole session with it on, preening and flicking his hair about. He'd regularly stick bananas up the kit man's exhaust; or would take the whistle off the kettle and attach that to someone's exhaust pipe too, so when you drove away all you could hear was a high pitched whistle!

Gazza would get obsessions over things. I remember at Everton he had this craze for having to do things in threes. One day he came back from the tattooist having had three tattoos done. He would come in and eat three bags of wine gums; another day it would be packs of ham, or tins of beans. Each time, he couldn't finish until he had eaten three of something. Then he would make himself sick and spew them up again.

In Glasgow, Gazza was the king. We'd come across him and the other Rangers players on our nights out. Gazza would call us over, and we'd go and have a drink with him. We'd sit down for an hour or so, and then move on. It was always quite friendly on a player level, despite them being the big rivals. That was probably more so for the English players – the Scottish lads would be a bit more wary, have a quick drink and go. But for people like me,

Gazza and the other English players up there, we were happy to have a chat, and save the animosity for the pitch.

That wasn't always so true when it came to the supporters. Glasgow was a great place for a night out, but as an Old Firm player you quickly learnt where to go and where not to go. I got to know that look, the one you got when walking into a bar and immediately being aware that you weren't welcome. The Scottish lads in the squad were helpful, pointing out which was a blue pub, and where was to be avoided. You either took their advice or learned the hard way. There were a few times when I'd walked into a pub and even before I'd got served, knew I had to get out quickly – occasions where you'd find yourself surrounded by a group of guys, ready to have a ding dong.

I never did anything provocative. I never went into any of those bars with the intention of winding anyone up. There were a few situations, definitely, where things nearly led to an altercation, but thankfully they never developed into one where it kicked off. There were a few times where I walked out sideways with some-one, basically to have a one to one with them, only for a bouncer or the other person's friends to pull them away.

That was Glasgow. There'd always be some guy who because he's had a few and is out with his mates thinks he can have a pop. As a Rangers fan taking on a Celtic player, that would earn him a few brownie points. You'd get comments all the time, people thinking they were big and clever, by shouting something out at you. More often than not, they wouldn't be prepared to follow it through. If you put them back on their toes, then suddenly they have a decision to make: do they look like an arsehole in front of their friends, or do they carry it through when mostly they don't want to? Usually, thankfully, it was a bit of bravado: the beer talk-ing. As soon as you confronted them, they shut up. The bouncers in the clubs were really good at dealing with it. Quite often, as soon as the Celtic players came in, there'd be two or three of them with us all night: they knew we'd be a target for some idiot, and so would be there to deal with it.

A lot of the abuse was wasted on me, to be honest. There were plenty of religious comments thrown about, and because I hadn't been brought up in that tradition, a lot of the comments went over my head. So they'd be saying something quite derogatory to me, and I'd have to go back to the Scottish players and get them to explain what it was the guy had just called me. There were quite a few situations like that, and I'd just laugh it off.

It was quite useful, in that situation, not being very religious. My family never had been particularly: we'd go to church at Christmas, and on similar occasions, but not every Sunday or anything like that. It was Church of England, rather than Catholic, mind, which could have been an issue had it got out. It was all quite hush hush: I don't think they ever asked me directly, but they worked it out without ever pushing too hard to ask what my background was. Certainly Tommy knew. The club wanted that all kept quiet – the line was that I didn't really go to church, which was true, and the press officer would dead-bat any other questions about religion away. They did that well, and the question never really came up while I was there – a rare example of keeping football and religion apart.

My first experience of an Old Firm game was one I'll never forget. It was at Ibrox and was quite early on in the season: certainly, it seemed to come by fantastically quickly. After the sending off at Aberdeen, I was beginning to find my feet in the Celtic defence. I was looking forward to the challenge, and ready to see what all the fuss was about.

I didn't have to wait long. I was still in the tunnel, preparing to go out to warm up, when before I had even got to the pitch I could hear a level of abuse that I'd never come across before. I'd been around long enough to think I'd heard everything an opposition supporter could shout at you. This, though, was something new.

'You Fenian bastard . . .'

'We're going to break your legs, you Celtic scum . . .'

'Hope you fucking get cancer and die . . .'

Looking back, there was something darkly prophetic about the cancer comments. That idiot supporter got his wish; well, the first part anyway. I was taken aback by the abuse and the sheer vitriol with which it was shouted. That, of course, was exactly what the fans wanted. As the team walked down the tunnel towards the pitch, the Rangers fans greeted us with a volley of spit. It was disgusting. I tried to duck out of the way, and had never been more grateful to get on to the football field.

I realised I had to get a grip, and quickly. We did our pre-match warm up, passing a few balls about. At one point, the ball got knocked off the pitch and I went over to collect it. There's a bit of room at the side of the pitch, a small asphalt track round the edge. I jogged over to collect the ball from in front of the advertising hoarding, and because I was right next to the fans it all started again.

'Fenian bastard!'

'You fucking Celtic twat!'

I was like, whoa! I got back on to the pitch before I heard any more, and made a mental note to keep the ball in play after that. It was one of those moments where I felt grateful that as a central defender I played in the middle of the park; it meant I was that bit further away from the fans for most of the match, unlike my colleagues who were down on the wing. It wasn't a pleasant experience, but it was good to get that all out of the way before the match started.

We went back in, had a final talk from Tommy and then lined up in the tunnel with the Rangers players to go out for the match. That was all right. The fans' hostility didn't make its way down to the players and the shouts were more normal: 'Come on lads, we're going to get stuck into these, today!' The comments were far more regular between the players, what you'd get in a tunnel before any match: there was no sectarian element or anything like that. For a second, you could almost fool yourself that this was just another match. Then you walked out onto the pitch and this huge blast of noise just smacked you in the face. The stadium had filled by now: we were surrounded on three sides by this sea of blue; then there was a fluorescent line of stewards, and a corner of green where the Celtic fans were. The Rangers fans were all pointing and shouting at us: the Celtic fans were doing an amazing job in singing their songs and applauding their team.

I could hear all the songs – the traditional ones that both the Rangers and Celtic fans sing. I didn't know them at first, but over the years I was there – I played in twenty-five Old Firm games – I got to know the words and what they all meant. That was certainly encouraged on the Celtic side. As part of the PR exercise of being a Celtic player, we'd go across to the supporters' clubs in Ireland, and be expected to sing these songs. The Scottish lads knew all the words already, but for the rest of us, there was a bit of learning to do.

The supporters do's were amazing functions to go to. I'd travel across to Ireland, and the level of support you received was incredible. The hospitality was always superb, and the supporters' clubs couldn't do enough for you. The event that always sticks in my mind was when I went across to the branch in Donegal one time. It was a big do, with something like four to five hundred people attending. We flew over and then I was driven down to the venue in a car. It was dark, and we were in convoy driving down all these bumpy, country roads. The guy driving the car was telling me it was fine, but I was thinking, just where am I being taken here?

The next thing I knew, there was this *'whup, whup, whup'* noise from above and a blinding spotlight in front of us. It's an army helicopter. We pull up and the helicopter lands. Before I know it, we're surrounded by armed officers and being pulled out of the cars and questioned.

'Who are you?'

'Where are you going?'

'What are you doing out at this time of night?'

I was shitting myself to be honest. It's quite an experience to have a guy point a gun at you, even though you know you've done nothing wrong. We explained who I was, and where we were going. The officers gave the cars a search and let us on our way. To go from that to the supporters' club was a surreal experience: everyone's singing the songs and watching you to see if you're joining in or not. This was before the peace process began in earnest, so it was still quite a sensitive time. That visit really gave me a taste of the tension, and the sensibilities of both sides.

That was the atmosphere in which the Old Firm games were played. We lost that opening game at Ibrox; in fact, in that first season, we lost all four Old Firm league games, only getting the better of them in a Scottish Cup match. The last of the league matches was the spiciest. Rangers beat us 1–0, but the story was really all about Paolo di Canio. Paolo, as I've said, was a passionate guy and having played in Italy for Milan and Lazio, knew all about the importance of a derby match to local supporters.

The atmosphere that night was particularly hostile. I'm not really sure why, but it was venomous, even before a ball had been kicked. It was one of those nights when football seemed secondary to the occasion. The sectarian element was right to the fore, and it was as if the fans were baying for blood. There were people in the stands repeatedly trying to get on to the pitch, and the stewards were struggling to hold them back. If the supporters didn't manage to get on to the pitch, then their passion certainly did so. First the Rangers striker Mark Hateley was sent off for head-butting someone. Then Malky Mackay got his marching orders. This was followed by a fracas between Ian Ferguson and Paolo: Paolo claimed that Ferguson had called him an 'Italian bastard' and was absolutely incensed. He'd got a yellow card during the match, but Hugh Dallas (who else?) was refereeing and after the game had finished, called Paolo into his office and gave him another one. Sent him off after the final whistle: you can imagine what Paolo thought of that!

What happened next was this ripple effect around the country. There were arrests after the match, about forty or fifty I believe, but because the game had been televised live, there was then this overspill of fans on the streets all around Scotland. Everywhere there were pockets of Protestant and Catholic communities, there was some trouble; flare-ups developed not just in Glasgow, but in Dumbarton, Bishopbriggs, and beyond.

As a player, it's hard not to let that passion get the better of you. You really have to work hard to keep up your normal levels of concentration, and not allow yourself to be caught up in the emotion of it all. Certainly, the referees, whatever their possible allegiances, let more things go in those matches, in order to try and keep a lid on things, and to try and keep enough people on the pitch. If they blew up for every foul that happened, there wouldn't be anyone left playing. I'm sure, too, that just as the players find it difficult not to get caught up in it all, so do the referees: sometimes it did feel as though they appeased the home fans, whether Celtic or Rangers, just to keep the peace.

I don't know what was said between Ian Ferguson and Paolo, but generally, as players, we were sensible enough not to inflame things in that way. And following the matches, especially if we lost, we didn't go out. The chances of meeting Rangers fans celebrating was a risk just not worth taking. We kept our heads down, and let them have their night.

The Old Firm game is something that the authorities have never really got on top of. Part of the problem, I suspect, is that a lot of fans come over from Ireland on the match day itself. So as much as the Scottish FA can try and deal with the situation in Scotland, there are all these supporters who are beyond their reach. From what I understand, the situation has undoubtedly improved from what it had been like in the eighties, but the problem itself has never been eradicated: what's happened instead is that they've tried to manage the problem. For much of the time that strategy is successful, but then there are games like that March one where it all gets out of hand again. Just before I moved to Scotland, there was an incident where a young Celtic supporter was stabbed to death by a Rangers fan after the match. He was only a young lad – an absolute waste. Football didn't save his life; it cost him his.

The Old Firm incident that everyone remembers from my time in Scotland was Gazza and his flute playing. That took place in a Celtic–Rangers game the following season. It was a strange incident, because none of us were really aware of it at the time: Gazza wasn't on the pitch but was warming up behind the goal. He did this imaginary flute playing, the flute being a symbol of the Protestant Orange Order, which was an incendiary thing to do in front of the Celtic supporters. But we were in the thick of the match and didn't even know it had happened. It was only afterwards, when the press got hold of it and the photos started circulating that it became this huge furore.

It was a crazy thing for Gazza to do. Knowing him as I do, I don't think it was done provocatively: he was just having a laugh.

He either wasn't aware or hadn't really thought through the sectarian connotations behind what he was doing. He hadn't clocked the potential consequences of what he had done – it was a spur of the moment thing, and I'm sure if he had his time again he wouldn't have done it. Anyway, there was uproar over it, and meant that the divide between the two halves of Glasgow became as wide as it had ever been.

The situation probably hit home to Gazza a short while later. He was in his car and stopped at a set of traffic lights when a motorbike pulled up. The motorcyclist knocked on the window, and Gazza being Gazza, he wound it down. The next thing he knew, there was a knife pointing at him.

'If you ever do anything like that again,' the motorcyclist told him, 'then I'll slit your throat. Understood?'

That incident alone tells you the level of hostility you were dealing with. That was a Celtic fan on a Rangers player, but it could so easily have been the other way round. That was how it was – a rivalry on a knife's edge, and in this case literally so.

It was a quite a first season at Celtic for me, though not such a memorable one in terms of club success. Rangers' dominance in the Old Firm games was the cornerstone to their winning the title, for the ninth time in a row. And although we'd beaten them in the Scottish Cup quarter-finals, we failed to convert that victory into cup success. In the semi-final, we were up against first division Falkirk. On paper, it should have been us going through to the final: when you play for Rangers or Celtic, you're expected to win every time. But on the day, things didn't quite work out like that. We lost – a match that turned out to be Tommy Burns' last game in charge.

Everyone was disappointed to see him go. Even the players who Tommy had left out were gutted by his departure. He was such a great guy, it felt hard to watch him take the can. To the players, he wasn't just a manager: he was a friend, a mate, he was one of us. Maybe that was why it hadn't worked out for him, but it meant that the affection we had for him was sky-high. We all wanted him to stay, and felt that if given time, he had it in him to turn the results around. Sadly, though, that was not to be. The man who'd sold me the idea of going to Celtic had gone himself. If the club were going to stop Rangers getting a record breaking tenth consecutive title, it would be under a new boss. And the manager the club chose for this task was someone none of the players had ever heard of.

# 7

## Champions of Scotland

*Wim Who?* That was the headline, and also the thoughts of the players, when the new Celtic manager was announced, just before the start of the 1997–98 season. All summer long, the press had been full of speculation as to who might be brought in, with high profile names like Louis van Gaal and Bobby Robson being linked with the club. The calibre of the people being mentioned was interesting, and was a mark of how the club's fortunes were beginning to turn around. The chairman, Fergus McCann, was not everyone's cup of tea, and he certainly had his moments with the dressing room, but from a financial point of view, there was no doubt he was taking the club in the right direction. After a sticky period, Celtic were finally on a sound economic footing – an achievement that, given the subsequent demise of Rangers, looks more impressive with each passing year.

It's easier to see that in retrospect: at the time, some of Fergus's decisions seemed only to rub the players up the wrong way. Jock Brown was brought in as a general manager, a move that didn't go down too well at all. While Tommy Burns had been a Celtic man through and through, Jock was seen as both a Rangers man and an SFA person. So he had his work cut out at the start to overcome this perception, and get the players on side. Doing so was a crucial part of the job – he was seen as the intermediary between the players and the chairman and needed to have the confidence of both for his position to work.

When it was announced that Wim Jansen was the new manager, I'd have to confess to being a bit nonplussed. We all were, really. Wim had pedigree as a player: he'd played for Feyenoord and was a member of the lauded Dutch team of the seventies. But as in the case when Arsenal replaced Bruce Rioch with Arsene Wenger, he had been coaching out in Japan, which in football terms was completely off the radar. Sometimes when you get a new manager, you know someone who's played for him before, so you give them a ring and find out what they're like. With Wim, however, we were all starting from scratch. And that was probably as true for him as it was for us.

The first time I met him, he seemed completely unprepossessing. He was this small guy with permed hair and I thought to myself, 'My God, who have they got here?' But it didn't take long for Wim to put the players at ease, and for us to realise that Fergus had unearthed a real gem of a manager. The thing about Wim was that he had this fantastic manner to him. He was quite quiet, certainly quietly spoken, but talked knowledgeably from the start; he gave off that air of authority without having to raise his voice to get it.

Wim had this strong Dutch accent that to begin with gave us the giggles. But what he was saying was exactly what we wanted to hear.

'Boys,' he said in one of his early sessions, 'we are going to play football. We are going to play it the right way. And we are going to play it to my way of thinking.'

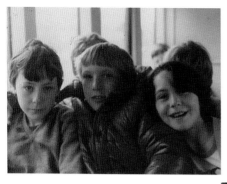

As a boy aged nine, with friends before a school trip.

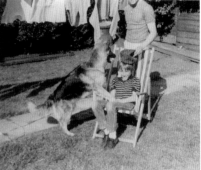

In the back garden, aged ten, with brother Ronnie and Sam, our German Shepherd.

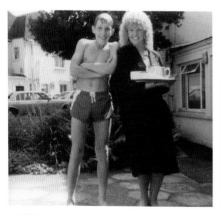

With a waitress, on holiday in Jersey, 1985.

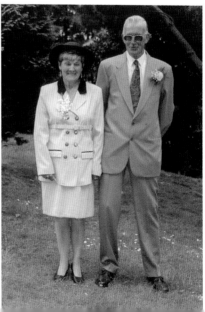

Mum and Dad on our wedding day in 1995 at St Chad's in my hometown of Kirkby.

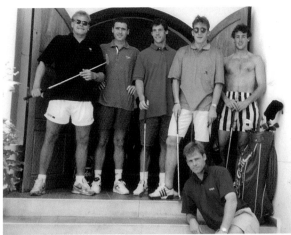

On a break with some of the Bolton lads in 1994. Left to right: Mixu Paatelainen, Mark Seagraves, Aidan Davidson, me, Scott Green and Neil McDonald.

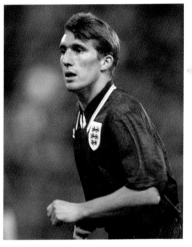

My one international appearance, England B v Northern Ireland B, 1994.

Winning at Wembley at last: Bolton Wanderers v Reading, 1995.

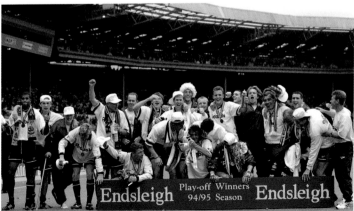

Endsleigh  Play-off Winners 94/95 Season  Endsleigh

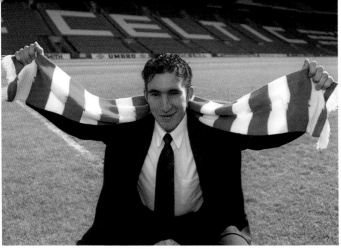

Signing for Celtic, 1996. The fee of £4.5 million was the most they'd ever paid for a player at the time.

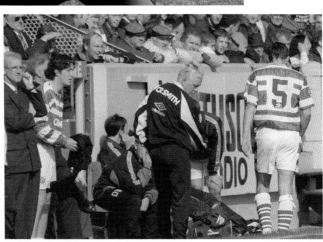

Not the greatest start: sent off on my Celtic debut against Aberdeen, 1996.

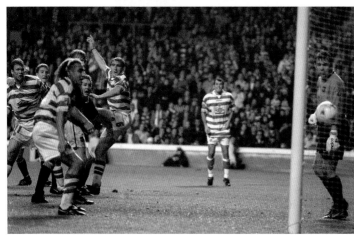

Scoring a late equaliser against Rangers: one of the turning points of the 1997–98 season.

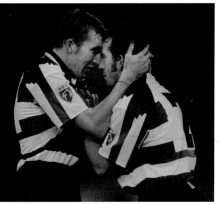

One of a kind: with Paolo di Canio.

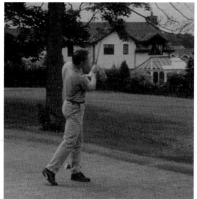

The fateful round: playing golf with my mate Stephen Deery and team-mate Mark Seagraves just before I got the call about the drugs test, June 1999.

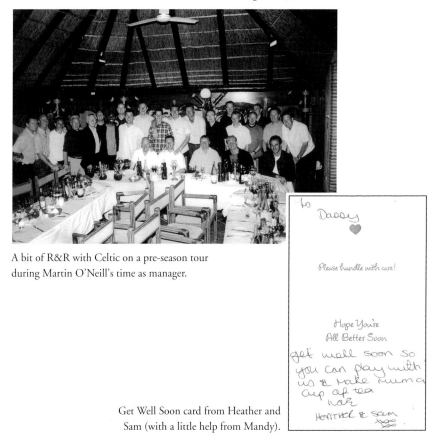

A bit of R&R with Celtic on a pre-season tour during Martin O'Neill's time as manager.

Get Well Soon card from Heather and Sam (with a little help from Mandy).

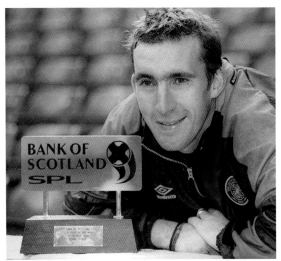

Winning the SPL Player of the Month Trophy.

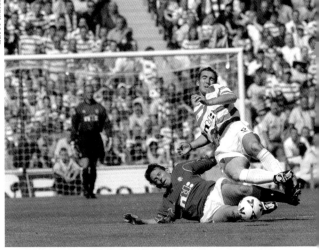

Tackled by Billy Dodds during the 'Demolition Derby', 2000: we went on to beat Rangers 6–2.

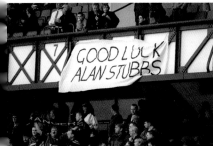

Old Firm united: a message of support from Rangers fans on my fight with cancer.

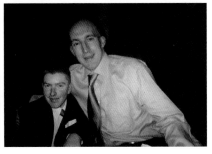

Fighting cancer for the second time (with Tommy Johnson's brother Wayne).

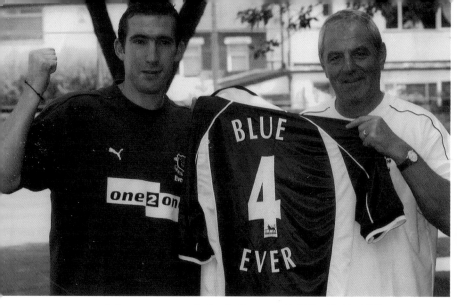

A dream come true: signing for Everton with Walter Smith, 2001.

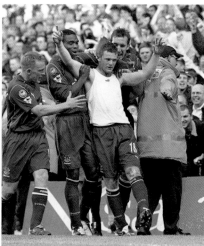

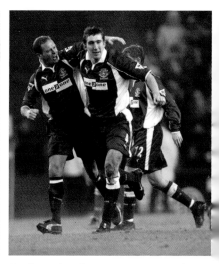

Celebrating another Wayne Rooney wonder strike against Arsenal, with Mark Pembridge and Joseph Yobo, March 2003.

On the pitch with Gazza: on opposite sides in Glasgow, together on Merseyside.

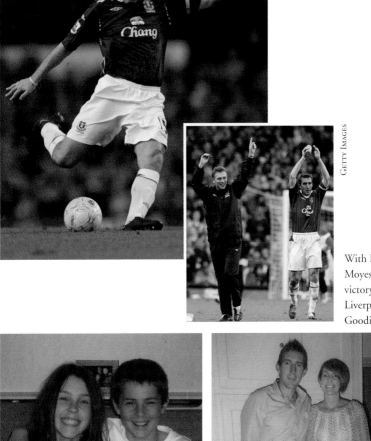

'Playing for Everton, winning somehow mattered that little bit more.'

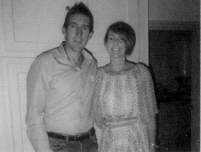

With David Moyes after victory over Liverpool, Goodison 2004.

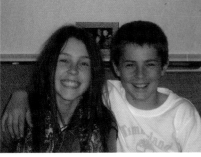

Heather and Sam, aged 12 and 10, in 2008.

Mandy and I before her 40th (sorry) birthday.

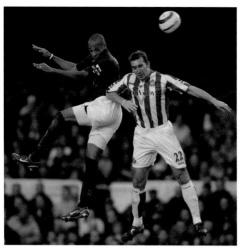

Standing firm against Thierry Henry during my brief time with Sunderland, 2005.

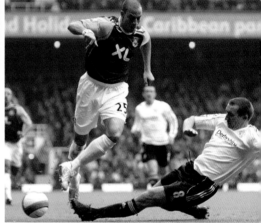

At full stretch against West Ham. Derby County turned out to be my last club as a player.

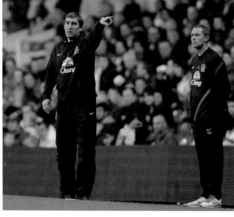

From defensive to coaching partners: David Weir and I both returned to Everton as coaches. David subsequently left to become manager of Sheffield United.

Thinking was something that Wim did a lot of. There was an almost philosophical quality to some of his comments and suggestions. There was one match early on in his regime, I can't remember against whom, when we had a terrible first half. We came in at the break and everyone was shouting and swearing at each other: 'Fucking hell lads, come on. What was that about? We're playing shite.'

Wim, though, was unruffled. 'Hey,' he said. 'Calm. Relax.'

He literally said a handful of words, but the way he said them just seemed to settle everyone down.

'A few minutes to yourself,' he said. 'I will speak to you in a moment.'

For some of us, this was quite a different form of motivation technique. I'd been with other managers where a bad first half meant fifteen minutes of 'fucking this' and 'fucking that' and ducking to avoid the crockery. But you know what? For Wim, it worked. We sat there quietly and waited for Wim to speak. When he finally did, it was like almost like Yoda was giving the team talk.

'You must not let frustration get the better of you,' Wim said. 'When you have frustration, you cannot perform at the best of your ability.'

Sometimes he'd speak like this and we'd give each other a look. *What is this guy on about?* But once you clicked with what he was saying, it actually made a lot of sense. It didn't take long for him to have us on his side.

Wim was one smart guy, a wily old fox not just in what he said, but in the way he dealt with the players. At the start of his time at the club, he put on what appeared to be some absolutely shocking training sessions. Just really boring routines that didn't excite the players: stuff you'd do with kids, really: running round with the ball, possession drills that were dull, slow and with no tempo to them. The players were thinking, why is he making us do this stuff? Does he even know what he's doing?

After a while, some of us started complaining. Wim just smiled his enigmatic smile. That was exactly what he wanted. He wanted to find out who the strong characters were in the team, who were the ones who were going to stand up and say something. So while we were all there, chuntering away to each other, he was building himself a picture of our personalities. It was his way of understanding people, and working out what made them tick.

Wim was also clever in how he dealt with the different culture of British football. He didn't come from a tradition of the players going out for a meal and a drink. Drinking in particular just wasn't the continental way. But rather than putting a stop to it, he allowed it to continue despite feeling uncomfortable about it, and despite us sometimes pushing the boundaries. There was one occasion where we'd played a match on the Sunday and Wim had given us a two-day break: we had Tuesday and Wednesday off, and then it was back to training on the Thursday. To cut a long story short, the players basically went on a two-day bender. We went out on the Tuesday and had such a good night we decided to have a few more on the Wednesday. A few quickly became eight or nine, and it wasn't until four in the morning that we got to bed.

The following day I got up at half past eight to make it in for training at half nine. The players all got in, but because we'd had so little sleep, and had drunk so much the night before, we were all still pissed. We started doing the warm-up exercises, and everyone was just falling over. Wim, who hadn't a clue what was going on, looked at us thoroughly bemused.

'What is happening?' He asked. 'What is this? What are you doing?'

He turned to Boydy, the captain, for an explanation. Boydy wasn't a big drinker himself: he'd have a drink, but not a skin-full.

'Wim,' he said. 'The lads have been out, and I think they're obviously still . . .'

At that point, Wim understood what was going on. It wasn't a situation that I suppose he'd ever had to deal with before in his managerial career, but I was impressed with how he handled it.

'Okay boys,' he said, clapping his hands. 'That's it. No training today. Go home to bed. I'll see you tomorrow.'

I can't think of many managers who would have reacted like that. Wim didn't read us the riot act, he didn't even raise his voice. Instead we got changed, went home and slept off our hangovers. The following morning, he sat us all down in the dressing room and gave us a talk.

'I understand lads,' he said. 'I know you go for a drink, I know you like to relax and enjoy yourselves. That is good. But it cannot be this way.'

We knew that. Everyone was really sorry for what had happened and we apologised.

'Okay,' Wim continued. 'No problem. That is fine. We move on now.'

That was all he said. The incident was never mentioned again, and it was never repeated. Wim wanted us to train well, but if that wasn't going to happen, he wasn't going to waste his time, or our time. Murdo MacLeod, who was Wim's assistant, would often take the training. There were times when he'd say to Wim, 'I think the boys are looking a little tired today' and Wim would just cancel the session: 'No problem. We do no training today'. It was smart management: Wim's softly-softly approach kept the players onside, but never at the expense of his authority.

That had an effect on the results on the pitch. There was pressure on the team that season to deliver. Everyone was aware that

Rangers winning ten in a row was a huge deal: for us it wasn't just about winning the league that season, it was stopping Rangers achieving that historic goal. Not that we needed any more pressure, but just to add to it, we lost a couple of matches early on. So right from the beginning we were on the back foot, which is the last place you want to be. Because Rangers and Celtic won the majority of their games, it meant that the Old Firm games tended to become more and more pivotal in deciding who won the championship. Once you're playing catch up, then they become all important. The other team know they just have to avoid defeat to keep their noses in front.

Wim, as you'd imagine, was quite unruffled by those early defeats. It didn't faze him, and he made sure it didn't faze us either. He wasn't the only new arrival at the club, and he knew that once the new signings had settled in, we'd have a really strong team. Over the summer, the squad had been strengthened by the likes of Regi Blinker, Paul Lambert and Craig Burley. Two crucial pieces in the jigsaw were incoming defender Marc Rieper and striker Henrik Larsson. The latter replaced the now departed Paolo di Canio, and it quickly became apparent the club had signed someone special. When he first joined the club, he was quite hard work. He'd been in Holland with Feyenoord and had the same touch of Dutch arrogance and self-belief that Pierre van Hooijdonk had. You want that sense of confidence in a striker, but in terms of getting on with them, it can make things a bit difficult. To start with, Henrik kept his guard up, and didn't really let people in. But slowly, the barriers came down: he started to mingle a bit more, and we realised that we didn't just have a great striker leading the line, but a fantastic bloke as well.

Henrik was one of those people who just seemed to be great at whatever they turned their hand to. A few of us were big golfers and he came along to join us. Before we knew it, he was getting lessons with a pro and improving leaps and bounds. He quickly grew to love Glasgow, and the green side of Glasgow loved him: Celtic fans adore their playmakers and their icons, and it didn't take long at all for Henrik to become one of them.

Playing against him in training, week in week out, was something of a challenge. Technically, he was such a good footballer. He had a good first touch, and had fantastic movement both with and without the ball. He had this ability of using his body to shift the ball one way and the opposing defenders the other. He was great in the air, too, especially considering his size: he was five ten, five eleven, but played like he was six three. Henrik had it all, really: he could finish with either foot, score with his head, but had good hold-up play as well. I was glad I didn't have to face him in a competitive match.

Marc Rieper was a key signing at the other end of the pitch: he was to be my partner in the centre of defence and together we formed a formidable unit. Big Rieps, as we called him, had come from West Ham and brought a wealth of Premier League experience to the table. He was a no-nonsense centre-half which was perfect for me. It meant that I could bring the ball out and play, safe in the knowledge that Rieps was behind me, covering my back. We had a brilliant understanding and formed a great partnership: one of the best of my entire career in fact.

The partnership I had with Rieps was replicated throughout the team. That season in particular, the players were always out together. It was a hard campaign, with a lot of pressure to perform, and we told ourselves that whatever happened, we needed to stick together. And we did that: we had a great team spirit. We had this saying that just seemed to stick: 'Smell the Glove'. It was a 'talk to the hand' kind of thing, meaning that we don't care what anyone thinks. The media can write what they like, anyone can say what they want. We are a strong unit and nothing's going to break that.

It actually became quite comical, the whole 'Smell the Glove' scenario. It became a story in the press, with journalists speculating about what it meant, putting two and two together and making five. At one point, a rumour went round that it was all about the Rangers goalkeeper, Andy Goram. We all thought that was hilarious. No one said anything, which just meant that the speculation and guessing game continued. Again, that helped us as a group, and drew us closer together: only we knew what 'Smell the Glove' really meant.

We didn't play Rangers until November that season. We should have played them in September, but the match was postponed after the death of Princess Diana. I don't think that delay hurt us: it meant that we had time to get our slow start out of our system. By the time we played Rangers, the team had very much became Wim's team, and had taken on board his methods and tactics. We played them twice in a couple of weeks, and the stakes were high: lose them both, and Rangers would be pretty much out of sight for the season.

The first match was your usual blood and guts Old Firm game, though thankfully without the edge and violence of the match the previous March. We lost 1–0 in one of those matches that could have gone either way. Really frustrating. Then a couple of weeks later, we had the chance to play them again, this time back at Celtic Park. To begin with, it felt like it was same old, same old: although they had Gazza sent off Rangers scored in the second half and seemed to be heading towards their sixth successive Old Firm league victory. If they'd gone on to win, it would have been bad, not just because of the points difference, but because of the psychology. Win and they'd gain that confidence from thinking they had the better team.

This time, however, it didn't work out quite like that. Our team spirit kept us going. We didn't give in, and in stoppage time we were pressing hard for an equaliser. I was up at their end for a corner and the ball came over to me. *Bang!* I put it away, and there was absolute pandemonium. It certainly wasn't the best goal I'd ever scored, but the reaction I got from it was immense. It was one of those goals that seemed to have more meaning to it than just levelling the scores. It absolutely lifted the crowd and at the same time knocked the stuffing out of Rangers. When the final whistle went, it was one of those draws that felt like a victory. We went on to beat Rangers later in the season, but it was that 1–1 draw which in a strange way felt the more important result. Come the end of the season, people were talking about how my goal was the one that won us the league. It had that level of impact on both the team and title race.

Following on quickly from this draw was the League Cup final. The competition was completed before Christmas in those days, and we were up against Dundee United at Ibrox in the final. That was a great occasion: we were firmly in control of the match, and ended up winning 3–0. It was great to get a trophy, and there were euphoric scenes afterwards, with everyone cheering and 'Roll With It' by Oasis blasting out over the tannoy. Coming so quickly after the Old Firm match, it just seemed to maintain the momentum, and continued the sense that we were on the up.

That was how the season continued. It was absolute neck and neck between us and Rangers in the second half of the season, but with victory in the next Old Firm game, it finally felt as if we had our noses in front. It ended up coming down to the last couple of games and could have gone either way. In the penultimate round of matches in May, Rangers got beat by Kilmarnock, which gave us an opportunity to finish it. But we could only draw at Dunfermline, which meant that they were still in it. We were down to the last day of the season, and one of those matches where the fans have one eye on the game and an ear glued to the transistor radio to find out what's happening in the other match.

Before the match, the pressure was intense. The build-up in the press was phenomenal, and questions were asked of us. Have we got the bottle to finish it off? That's where the team spirit came in: it helped us deal with all that. We can do this, we told ourselves, shouting at each other and geeing ourselves up in the dressing room before the match. Wim said the same thing, too, though in a slightly quieter, more thoughtful way.

It wouldn't happen now, but the final matches of the season weren't televised. They took place at the traditional time, 3pm on a Saturday afternoon, which made the occasion that bit more special for those who were there. We were at home that day to St Johnstone; kicking off at the same time, Rangers were away to Dundee United, a match they were expected to win. It was a great atmosphere at Celtic Park, as you'd expect. The fans were as nervous as we were, and it was a great relief when Henrik scored early on, in the third minute. That settled a lot of nerves. It took the sting out of the situation, made sure that it wasn't one of those matches where it stays goalless and the pressure starts to rise. There was still concern at 1–0: you're only ever a slip up from letting the other team back into the game, and in this case, letting Rangers back into the title race. Sure enough, the news from those listening to radios filtered through from the stands: Rangers were winning their game away against Dundee United. They were still in it: a good win from them and a draw for us, and they would sneak the title on goal difference. The game got a bit nervy, and St Johnstone got back into things: just before half-time, their striker George O'Boyle got on the end of a cross six yards out. It was a free header, but he couldn't quite keep it down and the ball, thankfully, skimmed over the top of the crossbar.

We were grateful to get to half-time. Wim did his stuff, calmed us down, told us we were okay, and we went out to finish the job. The rumours kept on coming through about what was happening with Rangers. But with twenty minutes to go, it all became irrelevant. Harald Brattbakk, who'd come on as a substitute for Phil O'Donnell, used his pace to get away from the St Johnstone defenders. Jackie McNamara, who'd been brilliant for us all season, spotted the run and delivered an inch perfect pass. Harald didn't even have to break his stride and walloped the ball into the back of the net.

That was it. At 2–0, we knew St Johnstone weren't going to come back. Whatever Rangers did (they eventually won 2–1) wasn't going to make any difference. There was still twenty minutes to go, but as soon as that goal went in, all the tension went out of the stadium and the place erupted. We were champions and had stopped Rangers getting their 'ten in a row'. It was an incredible feeling. Those twenty minutes went by in a daze: the game petered out as the singing and partying began. The stands were rocking, and in the case of the temporary stand while the stadium was being upgraded, literally so.

At the final whistle, it was just bedlam. Some fans piled onto the pitch. The players were all hugging each other. Even Wim was caught up in it: he forgot about his calmness and his philosophy and was waving and jumping about. The team had made 'Smell the Glove' T-shirts and we put those on: we knew how important that team spirit had been to winning the title.

Everything seemed to happen at once. We had the trophy presentation on the pitch, had the champagne out, had the photos taken. Our wives and children were there, and came out onto the pitch as well. I gave Mandy a sweaty hug and took Heather in my arms: she was only a couple of years old, so goodness knows what she made of it all. The crowd were brilliant, and we went over and applauded them for their support. They sang their hearts out – having waited so long to win the title, they were ecstatic. It was one of those occasions where with so much going on, you wished there was a way of bottling it up, slowing it down and stopping it whizzing past in a blur.

Back in the dressing room, the champagne was flowing. Everyone was getting chucked into the bath. We were all laughing at Wim, amazed to see him lose his cool at last, everyone enjoying the sheer release of the moment. Tommy Boyd went into the press room in just his towel to speak to the media. It was that sort of afternoon. And that was just the beginning. I had all my mates up from Liverpool for the match, and in the evening we all went out, players and mates. I've got to say, from what little I can remember of it, it was probably the best party I've ever had in my life. An absolute belter of a night.

The celebrations, however, were to prove shortlived. A few days after we'd beaten St Johnstone, the team flew out to Portugal for an end of season friendly against Sporting Lisbon. It should have been an excuse to continue the celebrations, but after the match Wim, back to his calm and collected self, told us that he was leaving the club. There'd been some sort of contractual dispute between him, Jock Brown and Fergus. I don't know all the ins and outs of it, but it basically boiled down to the fact that he thought they were taking the mickey. Wim wanted a new contract on the basis of having won the title: he felt he'd earned that, but they couldn't agree on an enhanced deal. The club wouldn't budge: maybe they thought Wim would cave in and carry on as he'd done before. Wim, though, was someone who stuck to his guns: he had his principles and had decided that if that was how they were going to play things, he was going to walk away. And that's what he did.

It was a sad way to end the season. The players had all grown immensely fond of Wim, and even if the chairman didn't recognise what he'd done for the team, the squad knew exactly what he had done for us. Within a couple of days, the headlines in the papers changed; from singing our praises, now all the old 'Celtic in Crisis' stories reared up again. I went off on my summer break, once again not having a clue who was going to be in charge when I came back, or what the following season might have in store for me.

# 8

## A Crazy Night in Zagreb

The summer after winning the title was a real case of déjà vu. Once again, the players had no idea about who the new manager was going to be. Once again, the media was rife with expectation: Martin O'Neill's name was repeatedly mentioned, which turned out to be a bit premature; Craig Brown was supposedly in the mix, as was Guus Hiddink. The rumours were so strong about Guus that at one point, the players thought he was going to get the job. Once more, however, the big names turned out to be just speculation and the chairman went for another slightly left-field choice in the shape of Jozef Venglos.

It was 'Wim who?' all over again. Venglos was a bit better known, due to the fact that he had been in charge of Aston Villa in the early nineties. But he hadn't particularly achieved anything there, and didn't leap out as a man with the potential to take Celtic on. Of course, all of this was true about Wim when he first took the job, and he turned out a success. So there was undoubtedly an element in the players' thinking of, well, the chairman got it right before, maybe he's got it right again.

Unfortunately, we soon realised this was not going to be the case. Wim was a guy you warmed to instantly, but with Jozef, right from the start, that same sense of chemistry wasn't there. He was softly spoken, exactly in the same way that Wim had been, but the warmth was lacking, and there was a feeling that he wasn't really communicating with the players in the same way. His English was okay, though not as good as Wim's, and he didn't have a translator. That meant that sometimes he was telling us things in broken English.

On top of which, the ideas he was trying to get across could be quite complex. Jozef's full title was Dr Venglos, and he came from a medical background and with a knowledge of sports science. As a subject, sports science was still relatively new at the time: the theories he was trying to implement were quite different, and took a bit to get our heads round. It probably wasn't the case that he was a bad communicator; there was undoubtedly an element of him trying to explain ideas that were a few years ahead of their time, and trying to get them across to a thick group of footballers who didn't understand what he was on about.

Some of the early training sessions he ran seemed to set the tone for the year. Jozef wanted us to be able to increase our intake of oxygen – all very sensible, scientifically, but not so easy to explain why in broken English. In order to help us achieve this, he'd have us running about and holding our breath at the same time. He'd have the stopwatch out, and make us hold our breath for forty seconds at a time. Then we'd stop on the spot, breathe out, and do the same thing again. You can imagine, as a group of players, we thought this was a bit weird. Wim had run some odd early training sessions, but he'd done so to check us out as personalities. There was method behind the madness, whereas here, it felt as though there was just madness.

Jozef's reign wasn't helped by a couple of other factors. Firstly, Murdo MacLeod, who'd been Wim's number two, had also been dismissed over the summer, so that link man between the players and the manager had been lost. Secondly, Jozef started just as the players were in the middle of an argument with the chairman, Fergus McCann, over bonuses. The bonus system was something that was agreed between Tommy Boyd as captain and Jock Brown as the general manager, the chairman and the senior players in terms of what we'd get for winning matches, trophies and so forth. It was something that was agreed before the start of the season and would usually be settled amicably and privately.

This season, the situation was different. Exactly as Wim had found when he tried to talk contracts after winning the title, Fergus would not agree terms to reward our success. The talks had dragged on over the summer, without reaching a resolution. The sticking point was over the bonuses for the Champions League. Having won the title, Celtic were now in the pre-qualification stages to get through to the group stage proper. That was potentially quite lucrative, and we felt a decent win bonus was reasonable as a result. Fergus made what he thought was an okay offer – which we thought wasn't – and he expected that to be the end of the discussion. Fergus was a hugely successful businessman and wasn't used to people questioning his authority. I think he was a little taken aback by how strong we were as a group of players – the team spirit fostered the previous season spilling over into these discussions. He didn't like that one bit. The senior players had a number of meetings with him, which were frosty to say the least.

We were quite determined, and told him that if he didn't budge we'd take action. We said we'd pull out of media appearances, things like that. Fergus was furious at that: 'Fuck Youse!' he shouted at us during one particular meeting, storming out. The last thing Fergus wanted was the situation to end up being made public. The Jock Stein Stand was now finished, completing the changes to the ground, and turning it into this incredible 60,000 capacity arena. The club had invited Liverpool up for a friendly to officially open the stand and Fergus didn't want this special occasion to be marred by the players refusing to speak to the press. It would have been hugely embarrassing for him.

The row rumbled on. It became public knowledge with the launch of the club's new away kit. Umbro, who made the kit, had arranged a launch and invited the press up, but when the day came round, the players who were meant to model the kit failed to show up, with the support of the rest of the squad. Fergus was absolutely furious: he slagged us off to the press, called us greedy and our position indefensible. Then, thinking he would punish us, he announced that he was deducting £50,000 from the proposed bonus pot, and giving it to a local hospital. Anything you can do, we thought. We trumped him by pledging that if he didn't play ball, the entire squad bonus would be donated to charity.

All this was going on when Jozef Venglos took charge, and it certainly didn't help his cause. Here he was, newly appointed, and stuck between a chairman who signed him and a group of players he wanted to win round. It was pretty much an impossible situation. He decided to keep out of it, which was probably the most sensible course of action he could have taken, but still it didn't go down particularly well with the squad. We weren't quite sure whose side he was on, and in terms of building a relationship with the players, it meant he got off to a bad start.

Despite all the bad blood in the behind the scenes negotiations, the launch of the Jock Stein Stand was a special occasion. It was one of those moments where you really appreciated the history of the club, and the long and proud tradition in whose footsteps you were following. The Lisbon Lions, the team who became the first British team to win the European Cup back in 1967, were all invited. I'd met many of them over my time at Celtic at supporter functions and other events, and they were always a pleasure to be around. Our kit man at the time, John Clark, was a Lisbon Lion, and he was always filling us in with little bits of history. Bertie Auld and Stevie Chalmers I used to come across a lot: Stevie was a gentleman, and a real character. Billy McNeill, the captain that famous night, was always around the club: he was a nice, really humble guy and would always stop to talk to you. He had his finger on the pulse, too, and really knew his football. In fact, the only key person who wasn't there that day was Jimmy Johnstone: he had beef with the club at the time for reasons I can't quite remember, and it was a shame he wasn't around. Whenever I had met him, he was always an absolute gentleman, and great company.

The launch of the stand reminded me again about how important history was to the club. This was something that as a new player you were encouraged to embrace. I knew bits about Celtic when I first joined the club, but not as much as if I'd been brought up in Scotland. I read a few books to familiarise myself with where the club had come from, watched videos of matches like that European Cup run: it was amazing to see the calibre of teams and players they beat to lift the trophy. That was really useful in terms of understanding both how important Europe was as part of the club's identity, and also the desire the club had for success. This was the standard Celtic aspired to – for the modern team to be talked about in the same terms as those earlier great sides.

The launch of the Jock Stein Stand completed the new look stadium: now the ground was surrounded on all sides, it meant that the noise made by the fans really enveloped the players on the pitch. The singing and chanting rebounded round, and made it a wonderful place to play your football. Liverpool were fitting opponents for the first match and they were spearheaded by one of the hottest young properties in the game, the teenage Michael Owen. Earlier in the summer, he'd introduced himself with the wonder goal he'd scored against Argentina in the World Cup in France.

Michael was a striker who was all about sharpness and pace. He was never going to dribble past you, but his burst of speed over a short distance was phenomenal. He was one of those players who, once he was away, you knew as a defender you were never going to catch him. He was still very young and quite raw as a striker, but that meant he played without any sense of fear. When you get older, and perhaps you've had a few injuries, you can sometimes feel a bit weighed down as a player. That extra bit of knowledge about matches and their significance can leave you worrying about what's at stake. When you're young, you don't really give any of that a second thought. He was a quiet player, Michael; not a talker like Ian Wright. He was difficult to read and was good at keeping back how he was feeling: a bit of a ruthless assassin.

Liverpool won the match 1–0, though there wasn't a lot in it. About as little, in fact, as there had been in the match-up between the two sides the previous season. We'd played them in the first round of the UEFA Cup, drawing 2–2 in a pulsating match at Celtic Park, and 0–0 in the second leg at Anfield , with Liverpool going through on the away goals rule. In the first match, Michael Owen had put his team in front: he'd given me the slip and then chipped the ball over our goalie, Jonathan Gould. We'd got back into the game and gone 2–1 up, only for Steve McManaman (just for a change!) to go on one of his mazy runs; he must have taken the ball sixty yards down the pitch before slotting home the equaliser. Even I had to admit it was a great goal. Although we lost the friendly, I was pleased to have kept Michael Owen shackled, and McManaman off the scoresheet for once.

The other pre-season friendly that was significant for me was when we went down to Bolton, to play a testimonial for Jimmy Phillips. It was the first time I'd been back to play since I'd left to join Celtic, and the club were now at their new home, the Reebok Stadium. It should have been a warm occasion – I had played at Bolton for eight years – but there was a bit of animosity remaining from some of the fans over my transfer to Celtic. Many were respectful and thankful for the service I'd given to the club over the years. But a minority felt I'd gone after the money, rather than staying at the club and helping them get promotion back to the Premier League.

I'd never seen it that way myself. I certainly didn't feel I'd jumped ship by going to Celtic. They'd done well out of me in fact, that £4.5 million transfer fee helping them to rebuild the team and win promotion again. But football isn't always the most rational of sports and sometimes emotions can get in the way. There are fans at any club who have brains like elephants: all they can remember is that you left them, and can't see beyond that to everything else you'd done for them. There's no doubt that players can be selfish, but the same can be said of supporters as well. Players want the best for them and their families; fans want the best for themselves and their club. There are occasions when those don't go together, and something has to give.

When my name was called out as the announcer went through the teams, I got a bit of a mixed reception: some fans applauded, but there was a smattering of boos as well. That hurt. If I'd been there and hadn't achieved, or if I'd left on bad terms, then I'd have said fair enough. But I couldn't really see it from their point of view. Fortunately, they were in the minority. And behind the scenes, talking to the board and staff, they were as welcoming and as pleased to see me as ever. I had a great relationship with them and still do: I could pick up the phone to them tomorrow, and talk away just like old times.

The big game at the start of the season was the Champions League qualifier against Dinamo Zagreb. We'd come through the first qualifying round against St Patrick's of Dublin, which had been fairly straightforward. Zagreb, though, was about as tough a tie as we could have got. At the World Cup earlier in the summer, Croatia had been one of the surprise packages, getting through to the semi-finals and only losing to the eventual winners, France. Their team featured six members of the national side, including the likes of Robert Prosinecki and Dario Simic. On top of which they boasted the Australian forward Mark Viduka, who would later come and play for us at Celtic.

Both teams were good enough to hold their own at the group stage of the Champions League and it was a real shame that we'd been drawn together. The first leg was at Celtic Park and made for a fantastic occasion. There's something about European nights at Celtic that are a bit special, and this was just as the UEFA Cup match had been against Liverpool the previous season, except more so. We had the new stadium completely full, and this huge prize of group qualification up for grabs.

The bonus situation was still dragging on – indeed, after the match, the players refused to fulfil their obligations to speak to the media. But we were professional enough not to let it affect our performance. I was quite glad, frankly, to be able to concentrate on the football again. Zagreb, it quickly became clear, were going to be a really tough team to get past. For me, at the back, I had a real handful to deal with in the shape of Viduka. I'd go as far as to say he was one of the most physical strikers I ever played against. Not physical as in dirty, but in terms of his strength. The guy obviously worked out and did his weights: he was a thickset lad, and when you went in to tackle him, you could feel the strength of his body. I had a couple of elbows in the face off him – accidental or on purpose, who knows? – and he had a couple back off me for good measure. It was a good, hard physical battle between us, and that was the way it was all over the pitch. We kept a clean sheet, which was great, and grabbed a winner, and that was fantastic. We maintained the long standing record of few teams coming to Celtic Park and leaving with anything to show for it.

Even so, the team were under no illusions as to how difficult the return leg was going to be. What we hadn't clocked, however, was the hostile reception we'd face when we went over there. The vitriol we received seemed to start as soon as our plane touched down at the airport. The Zagreb fans were out there in force to 'welcome' us, shouting abuse as we made our way to the team bus.

'We're going to kill you . . .'

'Tomorrow you die . . .'

Once we got to the hotel it was no better. That was a weird place to stay: it was full of prostitutes, quite openly going about their business. Extraordinary. The hotel became the focal point with Celtic fans gathering outside and singing, and Zagreb fans hurling their abuse in return. It was one of those occasions where you felt a little trapped. I wanted to go and get some fresh air, but the one time I stepped out of the hotel, it was clear immediately what the atmosphere was like. We had security with us, but even then there were enough unsavoury characters about that you didn't really want to hang around. It was all quite intimidating.

That theme continued on the way to the game as well. We had a police escort to the stadium, with officers screaming at the traffic to get us through. They wanted to keep us moving, because all the way along our coach was a target for the opposition fans: they were throwing stones, bottles, anything they could get their hands on. I was sitting on the coach and trying to laugh it off with my team-mates, but it was difficult not to feel a bit unsettled by what was going on. As we got to the stadium, there were hordes of Zagreb fans at the gates, singing and making this tremendous noise. I swear our driver, who was Croatian, drove as slowly as he possibly could through all of that!

We finally got into the stadium, got changed and went out onto the pitch to do a bit of warming up. Zagreb is one of those stadiums where you come up from underground, round behind one of the goals. While it's common in Britain for grounds to still be fairly empty forty-five minutes before kick-off, here it was already packed, and where the tunnel came out was very much the Zagreb end. It was a really unpleasant greeting: high-pitched whistles, booing, and amongst it all was the unmistakeable sound of monkey chants. It was like stepping back in time. I remembered hearing the occasional chant when I was growing up: it certainly wasn't a regular occurrence at Goodison, but I'd be lying if I said I never heard anything. But what I certainly never experienced in the UK was racist chanting on this scale – it was so flagrant and widespread, and involved a large chunk of the crowd.

It's difficult to be surprised as a player about what the crowd might shout at you. But even so, that was quite shocking. We went back down the tunnel and the chants got louder: we could still hear them down in the dressing room. We were all riled by it: as far as we were concerned, we were a team. It didn't matter who the abuse was aimed at, we were as one on the pitch and the disgust we all felt was palpable.

Did all of this have an effect on our performance? I'd like to think it didn't, though we didn't do ourselves justice that night, getting beat 3–0. One of the Scottish papers, which might just have had a slight Rangers bias, described it as the worst display in Europe by a Scottish team ever. I don't think that's fair at all. It wasn't our night, that was for sure, but you can't take away the quality of the opposition. The final scoreline was more to do with how well Zagreb played, rather than how badly we performed. Prosinecki, in particular, was unplayable that night. He scored a couple of goals and completely dominated proceedings. He was one of those players who smoked forty a day and could put in the late nights, but who got on to the pitch and pulled out a top drawer performance. He alone was the difference between the two sides.

It struck home to me, and as Manchester City's recent experiences in the Champions League have shown, that this was a competition you couldn't just expect to play in and make great strides at your first attempt. There's a whole different style of football to adapt to and get used to. European teams are better at keeping the ball than British ones: we feel as if we have to go from A to B as quick as we can. That has started to change a little: Sir Alex Ferguson has been a big advocate of that, openly saying he has two systems, one for the Premier League and one for European football.

You have to remember that this was the first time Celtic had played in the Champions League for years – the first time, in fact, since it had changed to its new format. If we'd been playing in the tournament for two or three years prior to the Zagreb match, I'm sure we would have handled it differently. We'd have had more European experience in the side, and been used to dealing with such hostile venues. We may well have played differently, too: there is an ethos at Celtic, and a desire, to play attacking, flowing football. That second leg in Zagreb, when we had a lead to defend, may not have been the time for such tactics. We went there still trying to play our football, and were probably too open as a result. But if we had gone more negative, we'd have been criticised for that, too. Sometimes, you can't win.

\*     \*     \*

Far from kicking on having won the league, the start of that 1998–99 season felt as if we'd fallen back. To make matters worse, Rangers had responded to losing the title by getting their cheque-book out, and bringing in quality signings like Gio van Bronckhorst, Jorg Albertz and Arthur Numan. And to top it all, we had bad injuries to deal with: Marc Rieper, with whom I'd built such a strong defensive partnership, suffered a bad foot injury that kept him out, and was ultimately to curtail his career.

As the season went on, the difficult start continued. We were knocked out of the UEFA Cup by FC Zurich and the tension was everywhere: there was an ongoing row between Paul Lambert and Jock Brown that threatened to spill over, and the police had to be called to protect Brown from furious fans wanting to vent their concerns. In the league, too, we found ourselves back in the position of playing catch-up to Rangers. By the Old Firm game in November, we were already ten points behind our rivals.

That particular Old Firm game was one of those occasions where the form book was turned on its head. Not only did we beat Rangers, we absolutely stuffed them, 5–1. Henrik was on fire that day, and got a couple of goals, but the real star was one of Jozef's more controversial signings, Lubo Moravcik. I think the press were critical of the signing because Lubo had played for Jozef before, so they thought he was just getting one of his cronies in. He'd been around a bit too, so some journalists wondered if he was getting on a bit; and to look at him, this tiny little guy, you'd never think he had the makings of a top player.

Lubo, though, was absolute class. Yes, he'd had a long career – he had been capped over eighty times for Czechoslovakia and Slovakia and been one of the stars of the Czech team back at Italia 90. But he was still a fantastic player, absolutely majestic when he was on song, as he was that day. He had great balance, a wonderful first touch and was sublime with both feet – so good, you were never quite sure which foot he was going to kick with. Lubo was an old style, silky winger. He wasn't one of those wingers who went back and forth up the touchline, not at this stage of his career anyway. But you gave him the ball, and he'd do his stuff: unlock and unpick the defensive lines in front of him with a pass or a run. It doesn't matter how old you are as a player: if you've got that vision, it stays with you forever. That Old Firm match was undoubtedly one of his days. He scored twice and ran the show. It was a real shot in the arm for the team, that match: it stopped Rangers going thirteen points clear, which would have pretty much been game over before Christmas, and gave Jozef a bit of breathing space from the criticism in the media.

The 5–1 defeat of Rangers, however, turned out to be something of a false dawn. Unlike the famous 6–2 victory at the start of Martin O'Neill's reign, the win wasn't a reflection of things to come, but more of a one-off. As hard as we tried as a team, we struggled to match the momentum we'd built up the year before. At the back, we weren't helped by Riep's retirement, or the fact that I was also suffering from injuries. I'd always been pretty lucky with my fitness, but that season I seemed to get niggle after niggle: nothing major, just groin strains and things like that, but they were enough to keep me out for a few matches, and made my season feel quite stop-start.

That season the groin injury wasn't really going away. Sometimes you get to the stage where you need a bit of help to get through it: to allow you to keep playing through the pain, rather than waiting for it to heal itself. I discussed this with the physios and they suggested that I have a steroid injection in my groin. This would decrease the inflammation in the area, unlike the tablets that I was already taking, and could get right into the particular area, and be more exact in where the treatment was working.

I certainly needed something. The anti-inflammatory tablets were masking the pain, but not sufficiently so. The injury was close to my core, from which comes a lot of your strength as a defender. It meant that I could feel it every time I was twisting or turning my body. I also felt it when I was running. All of which makes it difficult for your normal game not to be affected.

I should say that as always with physios, it is the player's decision as to whether to take the course of action or not. As at any club, the physio will make recommendations and suggestions, but there's never any pressure to make you go down a particular course. If I hadn't wanted the injection, I could have said so, and stuck to the tablets. But I was eager to get back on the pitch as quickly as possible. Part of that was because I wanted to play, but part of it was because I'm not great as a patient. I can't abide sitting still – the thought of lying on a bed for three or four hours not doing anything drives me up the wall. It might be the 'total rest' that an injury requires, but it always feels a waste of a day to me. If I was in the treatment room, I'd always end up being mischievous and playing practical jokes, or bunking off to watch the lads do their training.

So having the injection felt a bit of a no-brainer at the time. I didn't think twice about it, and was pleased that the pain had gone and I was able to play more freely again. It was only later, much later, when I found myself thinking about it. It was probably a complete coincidence, but it wasn't too long after I had the injection down there that I developed and was diagnosed with testicular cancer. I'm certainly not a medical man, and have no evidence to back this up, but it left me wondering whether this was the start of it all. It's just a hunch I have that somehow the two events were related.

*   *   *

I was back in the team, but that season it never quite happened for us. Jozef had more and more the feel of a stop-gap manager, and it was no surprise when it was announced he was being relieved of his duties. Jozef's wasn't going to be the only departure before the end of the season. Fergus McCann, the chairman, stepped down too. He sold his shares and took his leave of the club. In came a new chief executive, Allan MacDonald. In contrast to the barrier that had built up between Fergus and the players, Allan offered a more conciliatory approach and relations quickly became far more friendly. Allan worked hard at getting the players on board, and that was something we all appreciated.

That's not to take anything away from Fergus McCann and what he achieved at the club. He had taken over when the club was close to bankruptcy and promised he'd get it back into the black. He said he'd wipe away the debt and then take his leave. You can say what you like about Fergus – and plenty of people were not short of an opinion or two – but he was true to his word. Certainly, he could be ruthless in his business dealings, and everyone behind the scenes lived in fear of him, but he turned the fortunes of the club around. Effectively, he saved Celtic. As I said earlier, you only have to look at how Rangers' riches at the time have since unravelled to realise what an achievement his was. Fergus might have been a difficult guy to deal with on a personal level, but what he did for the club off the pitch was crucial for the club's success on it.

The end of the season was all about Rangers, and not in a good way. They rubbed our noses in it with their 3–0 win at Celtic Park, the result that won them the title. No one came out of that encounter looking good: the referee Hugh Dallas was hit by a coin, there were 68 arrests at the ground and another 45 in the city centre. Three hundred fans clashed in Duke Street, with bottles and bricks being thrown at police horses trying to control the situation.

Certainly, there were things that both sides did that didn't help the situation. Rangers mocking the Celtic team huddle probably wasn't the most sensible thing to do in the world. Equally, when our defender Stephane Mahe got sent off, he completely lost it and refused to leave the pitch. Stephane was a hard, no-nonsense player with a little bit of a short fuse. He brought the same sort of passion to the side that Paolo di Canio had done. On this occasion, he completely disagreed with the ref's decision, and allowed his emotions to get the better of him. Of course, looking at the situation rationally, when has a referee ever been talked out of giving someone a red card? But in the moment, that's not something you think about.

After Stephane's outburst, the sense of injustice on the terraces turned the temperature up, and made it all the more likely things were going to boil over. That's not to say there wasn't something in both Stephane's appeals and the anger being vented from the stands. It was another occasion where the whole issue of refereeing and neutrality came into question – you couldn't help escape the feeling that the referee was a Rangers fan and had it in for us. In a way, it doesn't matter even if there is nothing in the allegations – the perception there might be bias is toxic enough. Certainly, the following season Celtic wrote to the SFA and asked that Hugh Dallas be stopped from refereeing Old Firm games. The SFA, which had long been renowned as an organisation with a lot of Rangers fans among its employees, ignored the letter. And so the cycle of suspicion and resentment went on.

I've been in the game long enough to know that referees can sometimes seem a bit of an easy target: I'm certainly not the first footballer ever to have an opinion on how they run the game. But certainly in Scotland, and Hugh Dallas was typical of this, there was an abruptness to their refereeing style that didn't do them any favours. They'd be quite cold in their decision-making, dismissing you with a wave of a hand or a 'get away' and refusing to talk to you about why they'd blown their whistle. So it wasn't that they were bad referees in their decision-making, but that element of communicating with the players or explaining what was happening tended to be lacking. There was pressure on them, for sure, and especially in Old Firm games: there were certainly incidents where irate fans put a brick through their window after the match. They were well aware of the implications of making a poor decision or a bad call: perhaps that's why they were often tense and refused to speak to us.

Looking back over my career, I've always found that the best referees are the ones who are more hands-on with the players; the ones who would be serious when they needed to be, but light-hearted when the mood took them. So you knew where you stood with them, but could have a bit of banter with them at the same time. When they talk to you, you tend to feel more respect for them. I'd always much rather the referee said, 'Stubbsy, listen, you don't know what you're talking about' than just snapping at me like he was a school teacher.

It's a difficult job being a referee, I do appreciate that. And as the game has grown, and the money involved has ballooned, so the pressure to make the right call has grown. At the same time, the game has become quicker, which makes the ref's job all the harder. Take offside, for example: the speed of the players and timing of their runs makes it almost impossible to get the decision right with the naked eye. I do sometimes think it's ironic how the game has become more televised, with cameras here, there and everywhere, and yet the person who'd benefit from them most is denied the access to what the rest of us are seeing. The officials don't have the luxury of watching the incident again and again, in slow motion and freeze frame: they have one look at normal speed from which to make their decision.

I do think the governing bodies could help referees more. There's a stubbornness from UEFA and FIFA over bringing video technology into the game that I don't quite understand. Everyone knows the game is crying out for that, and I think that's probably the general mood among players and managers. We're only talking twenty seconds out to define whether a decision is the right one or the wrong one. Quite often you spend much longer than that for a player getting a ball back and lining it up for a free-kick; or when the ball goes back to a goalkeeper, they have plenty of time before they have to kick it back.

The announcement that there will be goal line technology in the Premier League from the start of the 2013–14 season is good news. I think that's the right way to do it, step by step. If that's a success, and I've no reason to doubt it will be, then video technology could be extended to other areas, such as major incidents in the penalty area or sendings off. You don't want the game to become stop-start and dominated by appeals, but that hasn't been an issue in other sports. In cricket and tennis, for example, there are a set number of challenges you are allowed to make. A similar set up along those lines would be sensible.

Another area where I think tensions around refereeing could be defused is over their lack of interaction with the media, and also with players after the game. For players, there's no hiding place after a match if you've done something wrong. You have to come out, face the cameras and explain your actions. If a referee makes a bad decision that changes a game, there's no interview with the media where he holds his hand up, and says, 'I got it wrong'. I know there are some referees out there who would be happy to talk to the press, and I think it would be helpful for them to come out and explain why they made their decisions. But because some of their colleagues feel uncomfortable about doing so, this blanket ban on speaking to the media continues. That's frustrating for players and fans alike. And just as with the contrast between the referees who talk to you on the pitch and those who don't, so I think that referees speaking after the game would gain them so much more respect.

It's not just referees avoiding the media that is an issue; it's also a shame that they don't talk to players or managers after the match either. Usually, the referees will go straight to their dressing room, speak to their assessors about the game and then they're off. The incident at Stamford Bridge after the Chelsea–Manchester United match, when the Chelsea players stormed into Mark Clattenburg's room after the game, was a highly unusual incident.

The only real contact and opportunity we get to talk to referees is pre-season. What usually happens is that a Premier League ref will come to the club, and talk everyone through the changes and rules that will be in force for the new season. So for example, if there is a plan to clamp down on diving, then they will show you a succession of video clips to give examples of what they felt was blatant diving and would warrant a yellow card.

Even then, you come away not being completely clear about what the changes are. Some of the new laws feel as though they are there as much to confuse referees and players as to help them. The way the offside law has gone is a case in point. It used to be black and white – either you were offside or you weren't. Now there are issues about whether or not a player is interfering with play and so on: that leads to room for interpretation and a far more fuzzy picture. Once you go down that road, then you're back to questions about judgment and neutrality.

At the Old Firm game at the end of the 1999 season, those questions undoubtedly reared their heads. A few weeks later, we played Rangers again in the Scottish Cup final, where once again we found ourselves second best and coming away empty handed.

But I didn't have time to dwell on the animosity and rivalry, and the season's disappointments for long. I didn't know it, but the random drugs test I'd had after the Cup final was to be the pivotal moment of the entire season – and one that was to shape my life for many years ahead.

# 9

------

# Super Caley Go Ballistic

The first time I had cancer, I was back in training pretty quickly. The time from the actual operation to being put back through my paces was only about six weeks or so. I treated it exactly as if I'd had a hernia operation. As it happened, I'd had a hernia operation once before – a double one when I was only a month or two old. I still had the scars, and when I had the operation to remove the testicle that was where they had gone in.

My routine of recovery was left in the hands of the Celtic physios. I started by doing strength exercises and gym work, focusing on the abdominal area. By the end of the second week I was back to doing light jogging, and then built back up to full training from there. I was used to the routine of returning from injury, so it was nice just to be able to slip back into that. It also gave me a target: I'm a restless person, as I've said before, so if the doctors said it was going to take me eight weeks to be back to full fitness, then I was determined to be back on the pitch in six.

For the first few days after the operation, it felt uncomfortable, just from the initial efforts of stretching and sitting up. But these were only small pains and bearable. I'd encountered far worse on the football pitch. The biggest thing to deal with was that from a male point of view I was a bit lighter: one testicle down, to be precise. I didn't want a false one put in and was glad I'd made that decision. I soon got used to the fact that my left groin area felt a bit numb. It would stay that way for the best part of a year. Only then did the nerves start to grow and I got feeling back again. That was a bit strange – sometimes, almost out of nowhere, I'd suddenly get a tingling sensation down there. Other times I'd have a touch around, and wouldn't be able to feel a thing. That was all to be expected: it was part of the recovery.

I felt okay about it, mentally as well as physically. This first time round, I never went through the process of thinking that I could have died: I was very much in the state of mind that I'd had a lucky escape, and everything was going to be fine. I never for a second worried that I wasn't going to play football again: the specialist had said from early on that it wasn't going to be a problem, and I'd been reassured by that. I also wasn't worried about where the cancer had come from: I asked about my lifestyle and if there was anything I could do differently, but the doctors were clear that there wasn't. I was fit and as a professional sportsman was in about as peak condition as you could get. I didn't smoke, didn't particularly drink and ate a healthy diet. I had just been incredibly unlucky: the odds were small, but what had happened to me could have happened to any man.

The only difference, really, was that I was a footballer, and as a result my cancer was public property from day one. That can be a bit weird, finding your health as a major news story. But in Scotland, if you played for Celtic or Rangers, that's just the way it was. The response from the fans, I have to say, was humbling and overwhelming. The 'Get Well Soon' cards and letters from fans wishing me well came in by the sackful. They came to the house, they went to the club and they turned up in their thousands. They weren't just from Celtic fans either: there were letters of support from Rangers fans, from general football fans in England, Ireland and all over the world.

I felt a bit uncomfortable about receiving all these cards. For all my shouting and leadership on the pitch, I'm actually quite a quiet, down to earth person off it. I felt awkward being thrust into the spotlight, and being the focus of everyone's attention. There was also the nagging feeling that I didn't quite deserve all the fuss: I never felt that I wasn't going to get through the testicular cancer. I might have been naïve in that assumption, but my belief that I was going to be okay was unshakeable.

As well as letters of support, there were others from people looking to me for inspiration. That was difficult to deal with, and I felt a little helpless in knowing how to respond. My cancer was one with a 95 per cent success rate of overcoming; what do you say to someone whose chances of living are less than 20 per cent? I'd get these amazing letters where people would describe their battles with cancers, and detail their troubles and experiences. It was humbling to read. With everything they'd gone through, and how comparatively little I had, it was hard to know what to say.

It struck home just how much people look up to footballers as role models. I got so many letters because I was playing for one of the biggest clubs in the world, and because of the high esteem the players are held in by the fans. There's a responsibility for the players to try and live up to that, and that was certainly true here. People were asking for help, and I did what I could to answer their questions. I couldn't always offer advice, but I could tell them how I'd managed to get through. To begin with, I tried to reply to them all, but in the end there was so many coming in, I couldn't keep up. Eventually, the club had to write back to some of the letters on my behalf.

I might not have enjoyed the publicity, but I could see that it could be used to good effect. Testicular cancer, particularly at the time, was not something that received a lot of attention in the media. Breast cancer, by contrast, had a far higher profile in terms of awareness. That's partly down to how men are: we can be quite ignorant about our own bodies and crap at going to the doctor about aches and pains. Asking for help or advice is just not seen as a 'man thing'. Men often feel awkward about talking about their private parts in a way that women aren't: women tend to be far more open and comfortable in asking for help.

I'd be the first to hold my hands up and say I was no saint here. I was a typical male in not talking about my health. It was a sad indictment, really, that it took something as severe as testicular cancer to make me realise this. But having a scare like that makes you realise how ridiculous that awkwardness was. I could see, now, how stupid that was, and also how potentially dangerous that male attitude could be. If there was good to come from what I'd been through, then it would be that the publicity my cancer had created could be used to get this across: if men could be a bit more open about their health and their bodies then maybe they'd be able to spot things before it was too late. The good news about testicular cancer is that there is a ninety-five per cent rate of surviving it, as long as it is found early enough. Those are pretty decent odds – and all for a just a little bit of know-how and regular checking.

I was happy if my scare could raise awareness and help others. I did a press conference once I'd recovered, and all the media who wanted to come had to donate money to cancer charities in Glasgow to attend. We launched the Alan Stubbs Everyman Cancer Appeal and immediately raised £50,000. I then got involved with Everyman as a charity: they had various events and fundraisers that I'd attend, and I'd do what I could to help in terms of publicity and getting involved.

That awareness was certainly apparent back in the Celtic dressing room. When I went back to training, the first thing a few of the lads said was, 'Come on Alan, let's have a look.' In a way I probably wouldn't have been comfortable doing six months earlier, I was quite happy to show them. I'd be in the showers, and the lads would ask to see my scar. Even those that didn't ask, you could see them having a glance across for a look. Some of them were a bit disappointed – 'I thought it would look a bit more strange than that' was a typical comment. But it was nice to get that out of the way and for it all to feel like everything was back to normal.

I was very aware that wasn't always the case. Sometimes cancer sufferers can be made to feel as though they're not normal – you can get that sense from people's reactions that you're different somehow. It's like you become part of a different culture: you're one of them, not one of us. Intentionally or not, when you get cancer some people can't help but treat you as an outcast. As soon as the word cancer is mentioned, and I still find this myself, the guard goes up with a lot a people. You can see them suddenly becoming extremely wary and self-conscious about getting into a conversation on the subject. More often than not, they're not being rude, far from it. They don't know what to say, and don't want to offend. They can be worried about what sort of emotional response you're going to give, so they shy away from speaking about it and change the subject.

Maybe I was lucky that my workplace was the football pitch and the dressing room. Changing and showering meant it was all quite natural for people to ask questions and have a look: it would have been a bit strange for that to happen if I had been working in an office. The dressing room, too, is somewhere

where there's no hiding place. You've got all sorts of different personalities in there: some people who'll take the piss, and others who you can have a serious conversation with. I knew the banter would begin as soon as I walked back through the door. In that sort of environment, there was never going to be any space for awkwardness to develop. Again, I know that I was lucky to have that.

I got a great response, too, when I started playing again. There's always a bit of chat and stick between teams, but no player ever went there with the cancer. I never had a single jibe or negative comment about it from a fellow professional, and I was grateful for that: it was nice to see how the mutual respect among footballers held up. It was probably just as well it did, to be honest. If there had been any comments, I would probably have ended up getting sent off. Behind the goals, the fans, too, were generally fantastic. There was a very occasional comment, some idiot calling me 'One Ball' or something hilarious like that, but if you get a crowd of twenty or thirty thousand people, there's always going to be one. It was such a stupid thing to shout: their brother, father, mother or sister could be diagnosed tomorrow, and then how much of a knobhead would they feel? Thankfully, the comments never caught on, and they quickly faded away. After a while, everything was so back to normal, it was almost as if the cancer had never happened.

With everything that had gone on over that summer, it was a relief to be able to go back to thinking about football again. It now seemed an annual occurrence that I would be getting used to a new manager: this was to be my sixth season in succession under a different manager. I'd thought that Jozef Venglos might have been the strangest regime I was to play under, but his replacement took everything to another level entirely.

When Celtic decided to get rid of Jozef, they decided to overhaul the structure of the club too. Out went the traditional managerial role, and in its place came the more continental system of a director of football, in the shape of Kenny Dalglish, and a first-team coach in the form of John Barnes. Kenny, of course, was something of a legend at Celtic: after an illustrious career both there and at Liverpool, he had gone on to great success as a manager at both Anfield and Blackburn. I'd been hugely impressed with him when he'd tried to buy Jason McAteer and myself from Bolton, so his arrival instantly seemed an astute choice. The decision to appoint John Barnes as first-team coach was more unclear: he'd been a great player, for sure, but was completely new to managing.

I'm not against the idea of this European style set-up in principle. While it is a relatively new concept in the UK, it has obviously worked as a model on the continent for years. The key to it working is down to the individuals involved; it depends on how well the director and coach get on. If they don't, there is always that potential for conflict. Equally, if the roles aren't clearly defined, then that can create tensions, too – if the coach wants to get involved in transfers, or if the director wants to get involved in choosing the team, then you're always going to have problems.

Neither of those were an issue in the set-up at Celtic. Kenny was quite clear that it was the director position that he was interested in, and throughout his time doing that role, he stepped back from the training side and gave John Barnes his head. Kenny did the transfers and looked after that side of things; John coached the team. The pair of them obviously knew each other well and got on, so on paper there was a lot going for the appointment. It was certainly a head-turning decision, and its high profile nature a counterblast to the 'Wim Who?' stories of previous seasons.

The Dalglish–Barnes appointment made great copy and the press were full of stories describing the duo as the 'dream ticket' to take Celtic back to the top of Scottish football. There was just one problem in all of this: John Barnes came to the job without any managerial experience. I don't know if he'd done any coaching before he came to Celtic or whether he'd studied for his coaching badges or not. Certainly, despite his job title, it was Eric Black, his assistant, who took most of the training. It was an amazing opportunity for John, for anyone who wanted to be a manager. But right from our pre-season tour, it became apparent that he still had a lot to learn.

One of the things you have to be able to do as a manager is to trust your players. If you don't have faith and belief in them, then you're always going to struggle. The pre-season tour took us to Denmark, and we were staying in an okay-ish hotel. It was nothing too flash, which is what you want for pre-season: getting your head down and getting back into shape. The only problem with the hotel was that the food they served wasn't up to scratch.

Perhaps more than at any other time of the year, pre-season is the time when what you eat is really important. You're working hard to get yourself back into shape after the summer, and it's important to put the right kind of food back into your body, to help you refuel. The food the hotel was serving wasn't great – the pasta was like rubber, the chicken was tough, and so on. We complained about it, but nothing was done. The players ended up sitting down for the meal at seven and pushing it politely round our plates. Then at eight o'clock, when we were free to do what we wanted, the players headed out into town to find a nice restaurant to eat in.

Everyone was thinking about pre-season and eating sensibly. No one was having a blowout or ordering anything greasy: it was all pasta, rice, chicken, fish, everything we should have been eating, but decently cooked. No one was drinking either – it was all orange, lemonade and coke at the table. One night we were in this restaurant, waiting for our food and chatting away, when John Barnes stormed through the door and straight up to the table, with Eric Black sheepishly following behind. John was clearly furious.

'What do you think you're doing lads?' he asked.

We explained. 'The food is crap in the hotel, boss. So we've come out to get something proper to eat.'

'Why didn't you say?'

'We have said. But nothing was done about it.'

At this point, John leant over and without asking, picked up Tommy Johnson's drink. Tommy was drinking lemonade, and John Barnes clearly thought there was vodka in it or something. He took a big swig from it, and put the glass back down on the table.

'What do you think you're doing?' Tommy asked.

'I'm just having a drink,' John replied.

'You were having a check, weren't you? You think I'm on the piss.'

'What is this?' The rest of us start chipping in. 'Don't you trust us or something?'

The answer was clear to us. At this point words were said, and only stopped when our food came out. By that stage, John could see that we were doing exactly what we said we were doing. He was clearly in the wrong and beat a retreat.

The incident in the restaurant was a bad start. The following day, a group of us went to see him – senior players like Craig Burley, Darren Jackson, Tommy Johnson, Jonathan Gould and myself. We told John straight that we weren't happy: we weren't teenagers sneaking out, but pros who'd been around. We knew what we were doing, and didn't like the fact that he didn't trust us. To be honest, things just seemed to deteriorate from that point on. We felt John didn't just not trust us, there was a general air of paranoia about how he dealt with the whole situation. He seemed to be convinced that everyone was talking about him and plotting behind his back when, in fact, no one actually gave a damn. Hand on heart, we weren't into all of that.

I think there was naturally an element of insecurity to John as a person, and the role at Celtic exacerbated that: it was as if he felt exposed because he wasn't sure he had the experience to do the job. As is quite often the case when people are insecure, they overcompensate to cover that up, by trying to sound more confident than they actually are. The result was that John tried to act confident but ended up coming across as a bit arrogant instead.

Now, I'd be the first to say that John was the most fantastic player – and that's coming from an Evertonian. He was brilliant during his playing days, and the way he dealt with the racism he faced during the eighties is a testament to the man. But by this point in my career, I'd played under a lot of different managers, and could sniff out fairly quickly whether someone was up to the job or not. I felt John just didn't have it, either in terms of his man-management skills or in terms of his coaching.

He wanted the team to be very attacking, which was great on the outside, but on the inside it wasn't working. You have to find the right balance, cohesion and team spirit in any system, but you could see it wasn't working on the pitch. The main problem with the system was the division it made in the team between the front players and the rest of us. We had Henrik, Mark Viduka and Lubo and into the mix came new signing Eyal Berkovic: that's a lot of attacking talent. Everything was about getting the ball to them, and preserving their energy. So when they lost the ball, rather than running back and helping out, John instructed them to walk back into position. Strikers aren't always the most helpful in coming back to defend at the best of times, but John's comments just added fuel to the fire. Now they had license not to help out. It left the rest of us under the cosh and feeling like a load of hod carriers.

That led to arguments in the team: we'd be shouting at the strikers to come back and defend, and they'd be shrugging their shoulders and strolling back into position. The group spirit which had been built up so strongly over previous seasons was in danger of breaking down: we were in danger of playing as individuals, rather than as a team. We had meetings where the back players would air our grievances, but it made no difference. Our job, it was made clear, was to work our nuts off and give the ball to the flair players.

Perhaps there was something in all this from how John had been as a footballer. He'd been an incredibly talented player, and I suspect there was an element of moulding the team in his own image: giving the flair players as much license, and as little defensive work, as possible. But it simply didn't work. Already well behind Rangers in the league, John's time as manager came to an end with the club's ignominious Scottish Cup exit at the hands of Inverness Caledonian Thistle – the match that gave the famous headline, 'Super Caley Go Ballistic, Celtic Are Atrocious'. I was injured for that match, so wasn't playing. Not that I took any satisfaction from that: it was a desperately sad night for the club. Inverness Caledonian Thistle were a First Division team at the time, and part-timers at that, so everyone expected Celtic to progress comfortably. Instead, in horrible, sleeting rain, it was the 4,000 travelling fans who had everything to cheer about. The first stirrings came when Caley went ahead after a quarter of an hour. Celtic came back straightaway, Mark Burchill levelling the scores a minute later and it seemed like order might be restored. But then Caley went ahead again, with Lubo scoring an own goal, and that was the way it stayed until half-time.

I went down to the dressing room and watched as John struggled to turn the situation round. It was a chaotic scene, to be honest, with lots of arguments and recriminations flying about. Mark Viduka was going mad and threw his boots away.

'Fuck yer mate,' he said in his broad Aussie accent, 'I'm not going back on.'

John was simply out of depth as to how to deal with that. Mark wasn't to be budged, and Ian Wright came out for the second half instead of him. It made no difference – just before the hour, the fact it wasn't to be Celtic's night was confirmed when Caley got a penalty. Jonathan Gould went the wrong way and Caley finished the game 3–1 winners.

Would John have been successful at Celtic if he'd had more of a managerial background? It might have knocked some of the crazier tactical innovations out of him, but I'm still not sure it would have worked: his subsequent roles coaching Jamaica and Tranmere Rovers did nothing to suggest he was adapting to management. It's not as if you can't go straight from being a player to being a manager, or that Celtic is too big a job for a new coach: you only have to look at the success of Neil Lennon to see that for the right man it's possible.

That transition from player to manager isn't for everyone, and some adapt to it quicker than others. For me, the experiences of playing under John Barnes was one the reasons I wanted to take my coaching badges before having a crack at management. When I finished playing, I'd only done my B licence, and wouldn't have been ready to take a managerial job. It is only four years later that I have completed my Pro Licence, which shows what a long learning process it is. I'd rather go into a managerial job with the right qualifications than to have attempted without and failed from lack of experience.

John Barnes lost his job after the Inverness Caledonian Thistle match, with Kenny Dalglish taking over the coaching duties until the end of the season. The first thing that Kenny did was to come in and talk to the players. That was a smart move – he has always been a player's manager and sat there and listened to everyone's grievances. That might not have meant he was going to do some- thing about them, but the very fact he was listening was some- thing. As a player, it meant that you knew your opinions were being heard.

That did wonders in bringing the team back together again. Everything Kenny did over those first few weeks was geared to getting the players to feel like a single unit again. He binned John's technical blueprint and simplified the tactics. He put out a team that was going to be difficult to beat and started from there. For pretty much the first time all season, the players went out and played for the manager.

Not everything Kenny did was successful. He took to holding his press conferences in Bairds Bar, a well-known Celtic pub on the Gallowgate, and at the Celtic Supporters Association. He felt the club had had a bad press, and this was his way of talking directly to the supporters. But it probably backfired a bit, and rather than encouraging a less hostile coverage of the club as intended, did little to bring the media round to his side.

On the pitch, however, there was an undoubted improvement. Tommy Burns was brought back in to help with the coaching, and although we couldn't stop Rangers winning the league, at least there was a League Cup victory to savour – another match, sadly, I missed through injury. At the end of the season, when Martin O'Neill came in, the structure of the club changed again, and Kenny left. But he's someone I'm still in touch with, and speak to quite a lot. He and his wife, Marina, have done an unbelievable amount of charity work in the North-West over the last few years: Marina overcame breast cancer in the mid-2000s, and they've worked hard to raise money for cancer care in the area ever since. I've always tried to support them, and go to as many of their charity functions as I can. When Kenny was sacked by Liverpool in 2012, I was straight on the phone to him, to say how sorry I was. He's a top guy, and I was pleased to have had the chance to play for him, albeit only for a few months.

Martin O'Neill became the sixth and final manager I played under at Celtic. Out of all the new managers appointed during my time at the club, he was the one who stood out instinctively as the one to take the club forwards. From the start, he just felt like someone who was right for Celtic. He had the right experience, had enjoyed success and had ties with the club that all augured well. He was highly rated for what he had achieved at Leicester City and was a popular choice among both players and fans. Finally, it felt as if we had the right man for the job.

Martin's temperament as a manager was impeccable. He took over in the summer of 2000, and when pre-season training started, a number of players who had taken part in the European Championships returned back later. But for those of us who were there at the outset, he began by giving us a rousing talk, about what he wanted to achieve at the club and what he wanted Celtic to be. He got the players to talk about why they felt the previous season had not gone well, and it felt a great beginning. Martin's passion for the job was clear, as was his vision. He was a man with a plan as to how he was going to bring success back to the club.

Martin was a brilliant motivator, probably one of the best I have ever played for. He was the type of person who would walk straight past you first thing in the morning, and not even acknowledge you. As a player, you'd be worried that he'd just deliberately blanked you. But then you'd see him again later on, and he'd apologise profusely, saying he was in a world of his own. That was him all over – Martin was a thinker, but at the same time he didn't miss a trick. He'd be exactly the same over contracts: he'd tell you he'd sort it out, and then you'd hear nothing more about it. Then three weeks later, he'd say sorry, and that he'd had it on his desk for the last couple of weeks, but it was ready for you to sign. He always kept you on your toes.

Martin had this way of making all the players feel wanted and special. He would sit down with the players individually before a match, just sit you down for a chat. Ask you about the family, how the children were. Something to relax you, and take your mind off the game. Then, just before the game, we'd be getting ready, putting on our shinpads, tie-ups, ankle strappings and he'd be pacing round the treatment table in the middle of the dressing room. He'd go round and round, his face a complete picture of intensity and concentration. You could see him gearing up for the team talk.

You'd all be sitting there, waiting, and *Bang!* He'd hit you with this most fantastic speech. It would be so fiery and passionate, it absolutely got you going, to the point where you almost had to be held back. He'd break it down to individual roles, tell each of us how good we were, and what we were going to do.

'Today Henrik,' he'd say, 'you're going to score a goal for us. You're going to get that ball and put it in the net. Winger, listen, you're going to have a brilliant game against the full-back. You are going to take him on, inside, outside, you're going to put the crosses in. Full-back, that flank is going to be your own, nobody is going to get past you . . .'

Martin would be so fired up as he told you all of this, it was impossible not to get fired up yourself.

'When we haven't got the ball,' he'd continue, 'we are going to get in nice and solid, hard to beat. We're going to get back into positions as quickly as possible. There's only going to be one word today and that's US.' The talk would be three to four minutes of information, and would finish with this sort of upbeat, rallying cry. It was just brilliant. He was an absolute master at it.

Martin headed up a three-man team who looked after us: his assistants were John Robertson and Steve Walford, and the three of them combined extremely well. Each of them had different characteristics and qualities that they brought to the table. John Robertson – Robbo – was Martin's right-hand man. He was the one who would check to see if there were any problems with the players and what he could do to fix them. Steve Walford – Wally – was so laid back he was lucky he didn't fall over more often. The contrast with the intensity that Martin brought couldn't have been greater.

Wally would take the training during the week, and he'd bring with him this relaxed, carefree style. He'd keep things simple and was great at coaching. I don't know how many times we trained on a Tuesday (Wednesday would be our day off) and Wally would say, 'Right, today we are going to fucking train for an hour and a half and then I am going to fuck off. I'm going down to London to see my friends and get pissed.' We'd all be laughing away at this, and if anyone asked if they could train longer he'd shake his head.

'One hour thirty minutes and that is fucking it. I'm fucking going in now, and you can fuck off.'

Wally would take the training during the first half of the week. Sometimes Robbo would join in, and he was brilliant: you could see that he was still a fantastic player. Martin would be around the club, but he wouldn't come down to the training pitch at all until the Thursday or the Friday before the match. We'd train until about 11.30 or so and then Martin would come down to the training field, watch the game at the end and would take us through the set pieces.

In terms of all the managers I've played for, Martin's set-up was unique – he was the only one who didn't get involved until so close to the match. His reign as Celtic manager certainly got off to a flying start. Right at the start of that opening season, there was an Old Firm game that would go down in Celtic folklore. We beat the reigning champions 6–2 in a match that became known as the 'Demolition Derby'. The result, and the manner of the victory, seemed to herald the start of a new era in Scottish football. While the 5–1 victory under Jozef Venglos turned out to be a bit of a false dawn, this victory immediately felt very much the real thing.

We had this amazing start. Chris Sutton, who Martin had signed from Chelsea for £6 million, put us ahead in the first minute. We'd won a corner, which Lubo had fired in and I'd knocked on into the box; Henrik had got to it first, but his shot miscued and ended up in front of Chris. *Bang!* 1–0. In the eighth minute, we got another corner. Lubo knocked the ball over, and this time it was Stiliyan Petrov's turn, heading the ball past the Rangers goalie. 2–0. Then a couple of minutes later, it was Lubo again, this time jinking his way past the defender Fernando Ricksen and setting up Paul Lambert. 3–0. By that point, the fans were in dreamland: eleven minutes gone and we were almost out of sight.

It said something about how rampant we were that Dick Advocaat substituted Fernando Ricksen halfway through the first half. That gave Rangers a bit more stability, but only a bit: Lubo and Henrik had great chances to go four-up that somehow just didn't go in. Then, just before the interval, Rangers pulled one back: Claudio Reyna's shot from a Rod Wallace cross squeezing over the line, despite Jonathan Gould doing his best to save it. 3–1. A couple of minutes later, it was Rod Wallace's turn to find himself on the end of the cross. 3–2? The Rangers fans were celebrating, but the flag was up for offside. So 3–1 it stayed and the whistle went for half-time.

We knew Rangers wouldn't take this lying down and would come back at us strongly. But it was us who scored first after the break. Henrik Larsson's first goal of the match was sublime: the ball went long from Jonathan Gould, Chris Sutton chested it down to Henrik, who left Bert Konterman for dead before chipping Stefan Klos from the edge of the area. 4–1. Rangers attempted again to drag themselves back into the match, and pulled another one back through a Billy Dodds penalty. 4–2. But then Henrik headed in another to make it 5–2 – and right on full-time Chris Sutton bookended the match with his second goal. Final score 6–2 to us.

It was a huge result. Two years earlier, we'd stopped Rangers winning ten in a row, and we didn't want them to start building up another run of back-to-back titles. With Henrik and now Chris in the team, we knew we had a formidable forward line – a real handful that any defence would have difficulty playing against. Chris had had a strange career: he'd started at Norwich as a centre-half; gone to Blackburn where he'd formed the 'SAS' partnership with Alan Shearer that helped them win the title; moved to Chelsea for £10 million and struggled to score. So when he came to Celtic, he was quite quiet to begin with, his confidence was down. But Chris was Martin's sort of player – he liked to play with a big striker up front – and Martin was probably Chris's sort of manager. He gave him his belief back, and right from the word go, it was obvious he was going to have a great time at Celtic.

The whole club was lifted by that result. For the first time in years, it felt as though Celtic were back on track. We had a fantastic squad and a great manager, and it really felt as if it could be our year. Unfortunately, my own battle wasn't going to be with Rangers, but my other main adversary. Within weeks of the start of the season, the cancer was back, and this time the situation was far more serious.

# 10

'We've found a small tumour . . .'

Apart from the original numbness in my groin, there had been no obvious side effects from the testicular cancer at all. I had a scan a month after the initial operation, and that had given me the all clear. The doctors seemed happy and the scans were reduced to one every three months.

It was strange – when I'd initially been diagnosed with testicular cancer, I was adamant that I was going to be okay, but every time I went for one of those scans I was absolutely bricking it. I always insisted on going on my own, because I didn't want Mandy to be there in case they found anything. I wanted to be able to do that bit by myself. I felt incredibly vulnerable about the whole situation: for all the doctors' confidence, there is never a guarantee that the cancer won't come back. That can eat away at you. On the day before the scan, I'd often find myself in quite a dark place. I'm not the sort to mope or stew on things usually, but I'd find myself thinking negative thoughts – what ifs, that sort of thing. Had I been feeling any sort of slight pain or tweak, my mind would put two and two together and make five. What if that was it?

I'd go to the hospital, strip down to my underpants and put on a medical gown. They'd give me this disgusting fluid to drink before I went in: it's some sort of dye that highlights the organs in your body, and has an unpleasant aniseed taste. I'd try and take the edge off it by adding a bit of cordial, but it was still revolting. Then I'd be put into the scanner for 45 minutes to an hour – the machine scanned from my neck down to just below my waist. I'd put some headphones on, listen to some dodgy music, and try to relax. More often than not, I'd fall asleep, and because the room was cold, would wake up shivering.

Getting the results would vary. Sometimes, the specialist was there for the actual scan and he would monitor the machine as it was taking place. In those instances, he'd say there and then that everything was fine. When the specialist wasn't there, then you'd have to wait until the next day – a nervy 24 hours, believe me. They'd usually ring the club doctor in the first instance, who would then pass the information on to me.

The one-monthly scan went to a three-monthly one, and then because those were okay, I was switched to a six-monthly one. Towards the start of the 2000–01 season, I'd gone in for the latest of these. I felt in good shape. There were no aches or pains that my mind could use to play tricks on me. I wasn't feeling tired or fatigued. All in all, I was in pretty good nick: Celtic were having a storming start to the season, we'd just thumped Rangers 6–2, and life seemed good.

The specialist was there that day, so I was expecting to be given the all clear and head off home. This time, however, I noticed he was looking at the results particularly closely. When the scan had finished, he came over to me.

'Listen,' he said. 'It isn't anything to worry about, but there is something that has shown up on the scan. I'm pretty sure it's nothing, but I just want to double check. Go home, and try not to worry about it. I'll be in touch with you tomorrow.'

Even though I didn't feel anything, I knew immediately that something was wrong. I just thought, he wouldn't have mentioned it if he thought it was nothing. I went back home and spoke to Mandy: I told her exactly the same as what the specialist had told me, that there wasn't anything to worry about. Deep down, however, I knew that something was going on.

The following day, a Friday, the specialist rang back.

'Alan,' he said, 'I've been speaking to a few different specialists about your scan. A couple of us have got a difference of opinion as to what your results show, so I'm just waiting for another specialist to come back to me, as I'd like another view. But would it be possible for you to come in?'

I went back to the hospital, this time with both Mandy and the club doctor. We were ushered in, where there were three specialists waiting for us. My specialist cleared his throat, and told me the news that I'd been dreading.

'I said yesterday that something had shown up on your scan,' he said. 'We've all had a look at it now and it appears that you've had a relapse. We've found a small tumour, right at the base of your spine.'

'Okay,' I said slowly, feeling anything but. Mandy, at this point, broke down. Jack, the club doctor, tried to console her. I was completely focused, and staring straight ahead at the specialist, waiting to hear what would happen next.

'We've spoken about the best way to treat this,' the specialist said, 'but before we go any further, I need to know what your thoughts are regarding children.'

I wasn't expecting that question. 'What do you mean?' I asked.

'I mean that in order to deal with the tumour, we are going to have to put you on a course of chemotherapy. That is going to affect your chances of having children in the future.' The specialist paused. 'So if you want, we can arrange for you to put some sperm away in a sperm bank, before the treatment starts.'

I looked across at Mandy, who was still deeply upset. 'What do you think?' I asked.

'No, no,' she went. 'We are happy with two. We've got a boy and a girl, a perfect family.' So that decision was made very quickly, right there and then.

I turned back to the specialist, and looked him straight in the eye. 'Right, come on,' I said. 'What have we got to do?'

The specialist was a bit taken by my response. 'Are you, er, sure you want to carry on with this?' he asked. 'Would you like me to give you a couple of minutes?'

I shook my head. 'Just give it to me,' I said. 'What are we looking at here?'

'Well,' the specialist looked down at his notes. 'The first thing we are going to do is to try and treat it with chemotherapy. We'll give you three or four courses and this could have a number of consequences. The chemotherapy will either reduce the tumour in size, it will slow the process of the cancer down, or it will completely obliterate it. We're hoping it will be the latter, but we won't know until we start the treatment. If it doesn't obliterate it, then we'd hope the tumour would be reduced to a point where we can operate and have it removed.'

'Okay,' I said. 'So when do we start?'

Again, the specialist was a little startled by my reaction. 'I'm sorry?'

'When do we start?' I asked again.

The specialist blinked. This obviously wasn't the usual reaction. 'I haven't even thought about it yet, to be honest.'

'Look,' I said, 'I'm not the specialist here. I'm completely in your hands. Whatever you want to do, whenever you want to do it, I'll do it.'

'Okay,' the specialist said, 'how does Monday sound?'

'Fine by me,' I said. And it was. I didn't want to hang around: I wanted to get the process up and running just as quickly as possible.

'Good,' the doctor said. 'Go home for the weekend, try and take your mind off things. I know that's easier said than done, but just take it easy. Then come in Monday, and we can start the process.'

Of course, while most people have the weekend off, for footballers it is the other way round. I guess I'm not turning out for Celtic tomorrow, then, I thought. But when would I be back on the pitch? When I'd been diagnosed with testicular cancer, pretty much the first question I'd asked was when I'd be playing football again.

'It shouldn't be too long,' that doctor had told me. 'You're probably looking at four to six weeks.'

That had given me a real boost – I'd had a target to try and get back to playing before the close season was over. Second time round, I asked the specialist the same question: when will I play again? Again, I wanted a date: something I could focus on, and spur me on to recovery. This time, however, the specialist came back with a different answer.

'I just don't know, Alan,' he said softly. 'We're just going to have to take things step by step and see what happens.'

That was the point in the meeting when it really hit me. Up until then, I'd been completely focused on finding a way through. What the specialist had said felt like a kick in the stomach. Oh shit, I thought to myself. I am in serious trouble here. I realised now that the first time round was to pale into insignificance by comparison.

First thing on Saturday morning, we drove back down to Liverpool to tell everyone. I hadn't spoken to anyone before the meeting on

Friday: if there was news, then I wanted to tell people face to face. We stayed with Mandy's mum, and she was really shocked but positive.

'Everything will be fine,' she told me. 'It will work out, I'm sure.'

I went round to see my parents and that was the hardest thing of all, having to tell my father. My mum was upset, but I knew she was a strong individual. My dad, though, I knew he'd find it hard. He was of the generation who didn't like to show emotion in front of other people. He kept it together and then left the room: he went and sat in another room by himself, which was his way of dealing with it.

It was a shitty day all round. I had phone call after phone call to make, ringing my brother, sisters and best mates, telling them the news. It was exhausting, but it had to be done. I must have spoken to over a hundred people on the Saturday and Sunday, and I could barely tell you a word that anyone said to me. I was in that much of a blur, that much thinking about Monday morning.

About the only person I do remember speaking to was Martin O'Neill. Jack, the club doctor, had gone back to Celtic and told them the news, but Martin still wanted to ring up and reassure me.

'I just want to let you know that everything will be fine,' he told me. 'The club are going to be here for you, no matter what. We are going to make sure that you get the best treatment that is possible, and that you are looked after as best we can. And by the way,' Martin added, 'don't even think about worrying about your contract.'

It hadn't actually occurred to me, but at the time I was in my final year of my deal with Celtic, and would be out of contract in the summer.

'That will all be sorted,' Martin said. 'I will make sure that's done, and you won't need your agent or anyone to negotiate: it will there, ready for you to sign, exactly as you want.'

It was a great gesture from Martin, and a measure of the sort of man he was.

The news of what was happening, meanwhile, was starting to leak out: having missed the game on the Saturday, people started asking questions and the story made its way into the Sunday papers. That meant more phone calls and messages of support, including some surprising ones. On the Monday morning, Mandy and I headed back to Scotland; Celtic had kindly provided a car to drive us back to Glasgow. We were heading back up the M6 when my phone rang. I didn't recognise the number but I immediately knew the voice.

'Stubbsy?' said a familiar Scouse accent. 'It's Reidy.'

Peter Reid, one of my idols as a boyhood Everton fan, had tracked down my phone number. I was completely taken aback.

'Listen mate,' he said. 'I've just heard the news and I'm really, really sorry. But you know what? You're a fighter. You're going to get through this, I know you will. Stick in there mate, and you're going to be okay.'

I'll always be grateful to Peter for doing that. He didn't know me that well, but he'd taken it upon himself to track down my number and give me a call. It was typical of him as a person, and I was touched. It meant a huge deal to me. It was a brief moment of light on that dark journey north.

At the meeting on the Friday I'd been told what I should expect from the chemo, but with everything else, hadn't really taken it in. I'd clocked the potential side effects from the treatment – nausea, diarrhoea, hair loss and so forth – but that had been about it. So I turned up at the hospital not quite sure as to what was about to happen.

The first bout of chemo took place over three days and was done on the NHS: the specialists had been clear that these were the best doctors around. They gave me my own room, however, because of who I was. They wanted to give me some privacy and keep me away from the other patients. As soon as I turned up, the first thing they did was to give me an injection to set-up where the drip from the solution bag was going to go: it's an intravenous connection, and they went for the vein right down the middle of my hand.

There was no anaesthetic, the nurses just numbed the area where the needle was going to go. God, it was a big needle. I wasn't particular someone who minded needles normally – I'd had enough injections over my career not to think twice about them. I tend to look away when they're going in, but once the skin is broken I'm usually fine about them. This time, however, I looked round and couldn't believe just how long the needle was. You could see the needle going right up. You're left with a tube that comes out and on the end is a little cap, ready for the solutions and the chemotherapy to be fed in.

The first bag came in, and that was a solution bag. It was clipped up onto the stand and came down the drip into my body through the intravenous connection. It didn't hurt, it just felt a bit strange. And cold – you got this chilling sensation running through your body as the solution went in. It took about thirty minutes for it all to go in, and when it was done, an alarm bell went off.

After the solution bag had finished, the nurses brought in the first chemotherapy bag. You could tell the stuff was serious from the way it was brought in, in a black bin bag: the light can affect it, so it has to be shielded. Which is fair enough, but it doesn't do

much for your nerves, seeing it brought in like that. The chemotherapy bag was attached and in it went. This time, it took a
couple of hours for the bag to be emptied. The alarm bell went
off, and the nurse came in to change the bag again. The chemotherapy bag was followed by another solution bag, to wash it
round the body, and that was the routine for two days: solution,
chemotherapy, solution, chemotherapy.

I wasn't the only one having chemo, so as I sat there, I could
hear other people's alarms going off as well. That seemed never-
ending – one or more would be ringing every five or ten minutes.
That happened constantly, not just during the day but right
through the night as well. The entire time I was in that hospital
was punctuated by this relentless ringing of alarm bells.

The chemo went on day and night and was pretty much
continuous. I had the occasional break, but it was only for an
hour or so. It meant you weren't really getting any sleep. You
might snatch a bit here or there, but your alarm bell, or someone
else's, would quickly wake you up with a jolt. It was draining: a
really exhausting process. But I was pleased that the threatened
side effects didn't materialise as they might have done: I wasn't
particularly nauseous, or anything like that.

Despite being given a private room, it was difficult to be in a
Glasgow hospital and not come across a football supporter. There
was a young lad, about twenty, who was also in for chemo, and he
was a huge Celtic supporter. The nurses asked me if he could see
me. They told me he was struggling to come to terms with his
illness and it would mean a lot to him. I said of course. They
brought him in: he was a nice kid, but in a bit of a state.

One thing I remember I did when I was gearing up for my
first course of chemotherapy was to read the cyclist Lance
Armstrong's book, *It's Not About The Bike*. I'm not someone
who's ever been a big reader, but Armstrong's book, about how

he overcame his own battles with cancer and returned to the top of his sport, I read from cover to cover. I found it such a moving and inspirational book at the time, and gave it to the young Celtic fan to read.

At the time, I had no idea about any of the drug taking, or all the revelations that have come out about Lance since 2012. Putting aside the ethics of all that, I just think it's a fantastic shame that a book which could have provided inspiration to so many cancer sufferers is now tainted and discredited. There's two Lance Armstrongs – Lance the cancer sufferer and Lance the drugs cheat – and the efforts of the former have got lost in all the headlines. But that still doesn't detract from what Lance had to do to beat his cancer – the effort he went to, and the strength of character he showed to overcome it. How can someone do all that and then turn to drugs? I just don't understand it. Here's someone who has portrayed himself as battling all the obstacles put in front of him to become the ultimate sportsman, and it's ultimately a load of bollocks in the end. The truth about what Lance achieved was powerful enough without the cheating and the lies. It's such a shame that has now got lost. Such a shame.

I could have taken drugs to get me back to fitness quicker and stronger, but the thought never even entered my head. I'm not going to sit here and say that no footballer has ever taken drugs – of course they have – but there has never been that culture in the way that there has been in a sport like cycling. I've never particularly been aware of stories or gossip about how such and such a player has recovered *remarkably* quickly from his injury. When footballers have been caught failing a test, it has usually been for recreational drugs, rather than performance enhancing ones: you can count on your fingers the number of times a footballer has been done for performance enhancing substances.

That's partly the nature of the sport: a race like the Tour de France is brutal, and recovery is everything. You've got to get back on the saddle, day after day, which is why something like EPO is so useful. With football, where you're playing matches twice a week, quick recovery is less of an issue.

Which isn't to say that footballers won't try different things and techniques to give them an edge: that's fine, as long as it is within the rules. We're of a culture where if one team have found benefits for the players from a particular vitamin supplement or protein drink, then everyone else wants to try it too. Some of this can feel a bit borderline if you ask me: the issue of blood transfusions has cropped up recently, with Tottenham using 'blood-spinning' – a technique involving platelets from a player's blood being re-injected into the injured area – to help Jermain Defoe recover from a pelvic muscle tear. Some of this can be a bit wacky: caffeine tablets, for example. There was an incident in 2012 when an England World Cup Qualifier was delayed by 24 hours; because several of the England players had taken caffeine tablets before the match, they had problems sleeping and were sluggish when the match finally took place.

When I was at Everton, Duncan Ferguson was a player who liked his caffeine tablets. They were quite fashionable at the time, and there was a bowl on the side in the dressing room, in case anyone wanted one. I remember before one match, he grabbed a load of caffeine tablets and shoved them all in his mouth: I don't think he really knew what the consequences would be. He came in at half-time on a right downer – the caffeine which had got him buzzing during the first half had all worn off, and now he was on the flipside of it.

I've never really explored any of that kind of stuff myself, but I've always been interested in different techniques to help me recover from injuries. I've tried Reiki, acupuncture and reflexology to see if they would work for me. On one occasion, I had a bit of a knee problem: there was a bit of bone bruising between the two joints, and because of the area it was very difficult to treat. Conventional methods weren't working, so I agreed to have a go at something else. I tried acupuncture, and it didn't do anything for me. I had needles in all over, and was a perforated tea bag by the end of it, but the knee unfortunately was no better.

Reflexology, by contrast, just seemed to do the trick. First and foremost, it was great because it relaxed me, and made me sleep for an hour while I was getting the treatment. And psychologically, I felt that it was working from the off: my mind just seemed to think, oh this is good. Having had the reflexology, my knee settled down quite quickly: within a week to ten days, it was clearing up quite nicely. Maybe my knee was at a stage when it was about to improve anyway, but in my mind I felt sure it was the reflexology that had sorted it.

Back in the Glasgow hospital, I chatted away to the young Celtic fan. We talked chemo, we talked Lance Armstrong, we talked football. I gave him the book, and told him he should read it. If Lance Armstrong had survived his cancer, then maybe we would survive ours as well. The lad didn't look convinced about that, but thanked me anyway. I watched him go and hoped he was going to be okay.

I finished the course and went home. Over the following week, however, I started to notice that my hair was beginning to fall out. There would be patches on my arms and legs from where the hair had come from; the bed sheets in the morning would be covered. I decided that I wasn't going to have clumps coming out and wait for my hair to go: I went to the hairdressers and got a number one, had it all cut off. I still wasn't feeling too bad, so when the next Old Firm game came round, I went to watch it on TV at a local health club in Newton Mearns. I went with Tommy Johnson, who was injured at the time.

It got to the end of the game, and for no apparent reason, I suddenly felt freezing cold. I realised that I was shivering.

'Is it cold in here?' I asked Tommy.

'Not at all,' he said, looking worried. 'Why, are you okay?'

'I'm shivering,' I said. 'Do you mind taking me home?'

Tommy was a gent, he put me in his car and rushed me straight back. My mum and dad were staying at the time, and as soon as I got in, I said to Mandy, 'I don't feel good. I'm going straight to bed.'

Mum and Dad were concerned, but I didn't want to alarm them. They came up with hot drinks and I tried to reassure them. 'It's fine,' I lied. 'I've just got a bit of flu or something.'

As soon as they had gone back downstairs, Mandy turned round. 'You can tell me,' she said, 'how do you really feel?'

'Absolutely awful. I feel terrible.'

At that, Mandy was insistent. 'I think you need to go back to hospital.'

She rang the ward where I'd been treated, and before I knew it, they'd sent an ambulance around to pick me up. I was rushed in, and immediately put on a drip. The nurses told me that because of the chemotherapy, my immune system was very weak. All I'd done was catch the slightest of bugs, but my immune system wasn't strong enough to fight it. They put me on antibiotics and kept me in for a couple of days, until they were confident I was better.

'You're going to have to be really careful, Alan,' the nurse told me. 'Coughs, colds, anything like that, you're really vulnerable to. You're going to need to really wrap up warm from now on. You can't just go out and see people like you used to.'

I had another meeting with the specialist after that, and they made a decision to speed up the chemotherapy. They decided, in the specialist's words, to 'go very aggressive' straightaway, rather than building up to it. That was because of my fitness as a sports person: while some people can have an adverse reaction to their opening bout of chemo, I'd coped with mine quite well. So my course was upped from two days to three. Throughout the entire chemotherapy, I wasn't sick once. The doctors were convinced that my physical condition had something to do with that. The main side effect I suffered was the hair loss. I didn't lose my eyebrows, which I had been dreading, but pretty much everywhere else: legs, arms, head, the lot.

Because the chemo courses tended to work on the same cycle in terms of weeks on and weeks off, you'd be there with many of the same patients who were there the first time round. I remembered the lad who was a Celtic fan and asked the nurses if he was in and how we was doing. They shook their heads. The chemo hadn't worked in his case; he'd passed away. That gave me a bit of a jolt. He was so young. If I wasn't exactly sure what was at stake here, then I was now.

After the second course of chemotherapy, the doctors scanned me again, to see how the tumour was responding to the treatment. The good news was the chemo had slowed the growth of the tumour; if anything, it might even have made it a touch smaller. The doctors made the decision to operate there and then. This was way ahead of schedule: on the original plan, I was lined up for four courses before the operation. But given the progress made, they wanted to go in.

The doctors explained the procedure to me of what would happen next. The person doing the operation was a renowned cancer specialist: he was one of the leading figures in cancer work in the world, and to my good fortune, it just so happened that he worked in Glasgow. He was a nice guy, and right at the end of his career. In fact, it turned out I was going to be his last operation before he retired.

'So I see they've given me something big to go out on,' he said with a chuckle when I met him.

I was glad to find myself in such experienced hands, especially given the potential risks from the procedure. The operation was lined up for a Monday in November, and as with the initial chemotherapy, I went back down to Liverpool for the weekend before. First thing on Monday morning, I was in the hospital and given various consent forms to sign. The forms said that if I died in the operating theatre, then there would be no blame attached to the doctors operating. To be honest, I didn't really think that much of it. The starkness of the language didn't hit home: I thought it was just a form. I wanted to get on with the operation and get it done. So I signed, trying not to think that my life might be on the line.

I was assigned to a nurse, who was going to be looking after me during the operation. She was brilliant, really good at relaxing me and keeping me calm. I had the drips put in and was prepared for the anaesthetic: I was quite used to all of this by now. I was in a side room to the operating theatre at this point, where they do all the prep. The doctor who was going to do the operation came in, all masked up and ready to go.

'There's just one more thing we have to do before we go in,' he explained, 'and that's to give you an epidural to help you with the pain.'

The needle they brought out for this was the biggest I'd ever seen. I swear it was about ten inches long. My God, I thought. Just where do you think you are shoving *that?*

'I'm going to give the epidural in your back,' the doctor continued. 'You may feel a little prick as it goes in, and then hopefully we can get on.'

They positioned me so I was sat on the edge of the bed, with my feet dangling down. The nurse was stood right in front of me, and I leant forwards with my spine arched, waiting for the needle to go in. Behind me, I could hear and feel the doctor having trouble. He was doing his best, but it just wasn't going in. I could sense the doctor trying to shove it in, could feel it grinding on my spine, on my bone. He was shoving me and pushing me, jerking me back and forth.

'I'm really sorry,' the doctor said at last. 'The needle isn't going in. Your spine and your muscles are just too strong. I'm going to give it one last go, and if that isn't successful, we'll have to go in a bit higher.'

I'm really gritting my teeth now. The nurse comes round and grabs hold of my hands.

'You all right, Alan?' she asked.

'Let's just get it done,' I grimaced.

The nurse squeezed my hands and I squeezed hers, as the doctor gave the needle one last almighty shove. No joy.

'I need to get this in, Alan,' the doctor said. So he tries another position higher up, and this time it works. I didn't really clock what the difference was as to where the needle went in; I was just glad it had gone in at all.

'Well, I hope that works,' the doctor said. Then before I had any chance to think about what that might mean, he said, 'Let's get him ready for theatre.' I lay back down on the bed, with the doctor looking over me.

'Good luck,' he said. 'I will see you after the operation.'

Those were the last words I remember him saying. At that point, the anaesthetic kicked in, and I was out for the count.

# 11

---

# Coming Home

Nine hours later. I was in what I later learnt was the recovery room. I was covered up to my neck in a big silver sheet, to keep me warm, and I was completely out of it. In and out of consciousness, talking away about God knows what, but it was making the nurse chuckle. I wasn't laughing, though. As I started to come round properly, I could feel the pain kick in. This was different: it was excruciating, ripped through me, by far the most horrendous pain I had ever experienced in my life. *I hope that works.* The doctor's words echoed round my mind. I realised then that the epidural hadn't done its stuff.

It had worked up to a point. Sure, from my breast bone up to my neck, I couldn't feel a thing. But that wasn't where the pain was, where the tumour had been and where the operation had been focused: that area from below my belly button up to my chest was completely unprotected. And it really fucking hurt. To the point that it was debilitating. I was lying there, unable to move and feeling completely useless.

The tumour had been at the base of my spine. It couldn't have been situated in a worse place. They couldn't operate through the back, so they'd had to go in through the front. In layman's terms, they'd opened me up, moved various organs out and to the side to get to the tumour, removed it, then put everything back in and stapled me up. The procedure was slightly more complicated than that, of course, not least because the tumour was sat right next to one of my main arteries. If they'd cut that, then it could have been fatal.

The pain that ripped through me was in a band around the centre of my bottom. It went from my back to the front of my stomach. I could feel the staples, I could feel my insides, I could feel *everything*. By now, the gibberish I'd been spouting in my semi-consciousness was beginning to make more sense. I started screaming and swearing at the nurse to get me some painkillers.

'The epidural hasn't worked, has it?' she said. 'I'll see what I can find.'

The nurse came back with something. I don't know if it was paracetamol or what, but it was completely ineffective. The pain seemed to be getting worse: it was almost as if someone was sticking hot knives into me.

By this point, I'd been wheeled round from the recovery room to intensive care.

'I need more,' I said to the nurse. 'I've got to have something. I can't deal with this.'

She set me up with a morphine pump. I was clicking away on it like mad, but of course, it only gives you so much every so often. I tried more painkillers and more morphine but they still didn't really work. Then finally, after about four or five hours – though it felt like much longer – I could at last begin to feel a bit of the pain relief kick in. For about forty minutes or so, it was great. It all just felt that bit easier. But after that, something odd started to happen. I couldn't feel the pain, but I also couldn't feel anything else. I couldn't move. My whole body had gone completely numb.

I shouted to the nurse to come over, or as much as I could, given I couldn't really move my lips. The only part of my body that appeared to be working as normal were my eyes.

'I can't move,' I tried to say to the nurse. 'I can't feel anything.'

'Okay,' the nurse said. 'You've so much pain relief pumped into your body that it has gone the other way. I think what's happened here is that your body has shut down.'

That scared the life out of me.

'Your body will re-adjust,' the nurse tried to re-assure me. 'It should all come back.'

I didn't like that 'should' one little bit. Lying there in the bed, feeling completely helpless, I seriously wondered whether I would ever walk again.

My concerns weren't helped by the fact that I had visitors. There was Mandy and a couple of my best mates who had travelled up. They shouldn't have been allowed in, but Mandy had spoken to the nurse and she said they could have ten minutes. It was one of those situations where it was great to see them, but it clearly wasn't so great for them to see me. I had drips coming from all over my body, heart monitors wired up, strapped little clasps all over my chest, not to mention no hair and this bloody great scar, or the fact that I now couldn't actually move. I must have looked terrible, and it was difficult for my mates to disguise that. I could see it in their eyes as soon as they saw me. When I've spoken to them about it since then, they all say the same thing: *We thought that was it. You just looked that bad.*

The numbness continued. It went on for the rest of that day, throughout the night and on into the next. The night was the worst. That was when dark thoughts really tried to take hold. But the following day I woke up and to my delight, I could feel my big toe. I could wiggle it and feel it move. It was one of the greatest feelings of my life. It's coming back, I thought. And over the following minutes and hours, sensation started to work its way back up through my body, from my feet upwards. It was the sort of simple thing you wouldn't normally think twice about, but feeling it returning was amazing.

I was in intensive care for three days in all. On the third day, I managed to sit on the side of the bed and attempted to take a few small steps. The nurses couldn't believe that. They told me that anyone who'd been through the sort of operation I'd had wouldn't normally get out of bed for at least ten days. I started to progress: the next thing I managed was to make my way to the shower room with the help of the nurse. There was a chair here that you could sit on to wash yourself, but I was determined to be able to bend down and try and touch my toes.

After six days, I was released from hospital. Again, this was something almost unheard of. I was way ahead of schedule, but the doctors felt I'd be better off in the hands of the physios. As far as we are concerned, they told me, that is you all done. They'd never dealt with a footballer before, so it made sense for my rehab to take place back at the club. I was relieved to be out of there and once more determined to be back on a football pitch just as soon as I could.

My battle with cancer was a far more private affair, the second time round. With the initial testicular cancer, because of the drugs test and everything, it was big news: one of the papers had even run a story suggesting I'd failed the drugs test, without being in knowledge of all the facts. Second time round, because it was more serious, I think people gave me a bit more space. There was a lot more respect in terms of my family and our privacy: the press were a lot more professional on this occasion.

I still got plenty of letters: people would write to me who were either dealing with cancer or knew someone who was trying to cope with it, and ask me for my advice. I still found that a difficult thing to do – everyone's situation is different, and everyone is different, too, in how they come to terms with it – but I understood more from that second experience.

I don't think anyone knows quite how they are going to deal with cancer until the moment you are diagnosed. Even the second before, you don't really know. Once you are diagnosed, however, then everything changes. Suddenly it's there, inside you, this *thing*. For me, the way I dealt with it was down to the sort of person I am. I'm the sort of character that whether it's a situation on the football field or on a hospital ward, I want to fight it head on. I didn't know whether I would come through it, but I sure as hell wasn't going to just lay down and give in to it. If I was to go, I was going to go down with all guns blazing.

I was positive about the situation right from the off, and though I don't know how much impact that had, it certainly can't have hurt my chances. Cancer takes you to a place that you wouldn't wish for anyone to find themselves in. Some people's reaction, like mine, is to fight: for others, their response is to prepare for the end. Once you start thinking like that, then you're already on the slope to giving in.

I didn't make any preparations for dying. My will had been done years before and I didn't go back and look at it. I didn't think about funeral arrangements, or writing letters to people, making any videos or tapes or anything like that. I didn't want to entertain any negative thoughts like that whatsoever. I was determined to be positive. I'm going to beat this thing, I told myself, so why would I bother with all that?

When people said to me how unlucky I was, I used to laugh. Unlucky? I was the luckiest person alive. Would I have found that lump if it hadn't been for the random drugs test? I'm not sure I would have done. And even if I had, I'm not sure I would have had the courage to go and see someone about it. I'd had a relapse but I'd fallen on my feet in terms of the people who were looking after me: I was in the best hands that I could possibly be in. What more could you ask for? I had survived. I was in the lucky club.

I've been clear for over ten years now: that is the point when you are officially clean and free of it. The records might say that, but I don't think that you ever are free. I think cancer will always be part of you. I wouldn't say that I never think about it, but it's not something I dwell on. One of the things I've discovered about cancer, and coming through such an experience, is that it changes the way that you look at the world. I don't think you have fears and concerns about life in quite the same way.

Has the experience made me a better person? I would like to think that it has. It has certainly made me more carefree. Mandy would hate me for saying this, and I'm sure it annoys her some-times, but I live my life a lot more day by day now. What is the point in worrying about things that might never happen? This was something I decided when I was given the all clear. I thought to myself, okay, this is how I am going to look at things going forwards. I'm not going to sit here worrying about what if the cancer came back tomorrow.

I worry about different things, not so much about me. I worry about the lads that I train: I worry about what they are doing away from football. I worry about how I serve them and how I can become better as a coach and eventually, hopefully, as a manager. That all comes from care – if you care about anything in life, then you worry: if you don't worry, then you probably don't care. I'd far rather worry about someone I care about here and now. Rather that, than a hypothetical situation in the future.

The cancer changed my relationship with football as well. Before it happened, football was everything to me. Afterwards, football was still a huge part of my life, but it wasn't everything in quite the same way. My immediate family, my wife and children, parents and siblings, they were more important. I was still as fierce a competitor as ever on the pitch – I never lost that burning hatred of getting beat – but now, once the match was over and I was off the pitch, that was it as far I was concerned. I could call someone every name under the sun on the pitch, but now I could shake his hand and have a drink with him in the bar afterwards.

It was no small job getting back up to full fitness. The wound I had from the operation was substantial. It went down in a straight line from underneath my rib cage, a little kink round my belly button and then back down again to just above my lower belly. It was so big, they'd had to staple it over forty times after the operation. I've still got the scar today. In terms of playing football, the wound had a big impact on my game. All your main movements come from your core, so any type of twisting and turning during a game and you'd immediately feel it and wince.

I was put in the capable hands of Brian Scott, the Celtic physio. I've worked with some good physios in my career, but Scottie for me was probably the best. He was someone who was very good with his hands – he had this way of feeling your injuries and being able to put his finger on exactly the spot where you were having a problem. That's a bit of a dying art – modern physios tend to be a bit less active because of all the machinery they have at their disposal. These days, as soon as you are injured, you're immediately whisked off for a scan. Sometimes it can seem as though everyone is scanned the whole time, whatever the complaint.

For all my desire to get back, Scottie wanted to take things slowly at first.

'Go home and rest,' he told me. 'You can do a bit of walking but be very careful not to overdo it.'

Having worked with me for years, Scottie knew exactly what I was like.

'No overstretching,' he continued. 'No lifting, anything like that.'

I stayed home for about a week. I took it easy, as best I could, and started to sleep a bit better. After a week, I started going into the training ground. I'd go in two or three times a week and get exercises to do from Scottie: routines I could do both at the training ground and also back at home. It was all quite basic stuff to begin with – a little bit of lifting weights, or ticking over on an exercise bike to get my legs going. To begin with, the agreement was that as soon as I felt any discomfort, I was to stop straightaway.

Scottie didn't want to do too much on my core to begin with, because my stomach was still healing. I still had my staples in, and only had them taken out after a couple of weeks. It was one of those removals where there's a little silver tray at the side of the bed, and you could hear a metallic clank every time one of the staples was dropped in. There were one or two that made me wince as they were taken out, but on the whole, they were okay.

Slowly, and carefully, Scottie built up my exercise routine. We started to work on the core: a little bit of pain was okay, we decided, as long as it was bearable. I worked hard on core stability and did a lot of time on the bag – gradually building my strength back up and getting my cardio going again. By week four, I was back to light jogging. From here, I was at the point of starting the equivalent of pre-season training again – essentially, it was another eight weeks to get myself back up to full fitness and in a position to go back into full training. Not that Scottie and I ever really talked dates. Scottie didn't want to put any pressure on by suggesting a specific goal: it was all uncharted territory for him, and neither of us knew if there'd be setbacks along the way. He told me that if everything went well, then I might be looking to go back into training around this date, but made it clear we were taking things step by step. Scottie knew that if he gave me a set date to work towards, I'd try and beat it and that probably wasn't the best for my recuperation. He was probably right to do so. As it was, I was holding back on telling him how bad I was feeling at times, so desperate was I to get back onto a football pitch.

Even if I wasn't in full training, it was nice to be back at the training ground and around the other players. As with when I came back from the testicular cancer, there were no kid gloves and the lads treated me as normal.

'Here he comes,' they joked when they saw me. 'I suppose he'll be expecting the sympathy vote now.'

'Go and try your luck with the Gaffer,' the banter continued. 'You won't get any slack from Martin, just cos you've had an operation.'

Exactly as with the testicular cancer, everyone wanted a look. As soon I lifted my top up and they saw the scar, the reaction was 'Bloody hell, Stubbs!' I guess I'd got used to it, but when people saw the scar for the first time, it reminded me how what I'd gone through was such a big deal.

The Gaffer, meanwhile, was great with me throughout. The fact that Martin said what he had about my contract at the outset had been incredibly reassuring: it meant that during my recovery, I never for one moment found myself thinking, I've got to get back as quickly as possible or I won't get a new deal. It meant I could focus all my energy on recovery, rather than worrying about money and the future. Throughout my rehabilitation, he'd be on the phone or coming round the house to see me. Right from the start, he told me that I could come back to training any time I liked. He told me to come in and see the players whenever I wanted. He wasn't my manager through this process, he was a friend, and that was the best thing about it.

The Celtic physios were to work me hard, but not as hard as I worked myself. The team was doing well and I was determined to be back and part of it. I was so determined to get back and playing that I talked down the pain. I knew I was coming back too early – by about six weeks to two months, I reckoned – but I was determined to return. After everything I'd been through, I wanted to prove – to myself, as much as anyone else – that I could still compete, and at the highest level. So even though I wasn't, I told the physios I was okay, and ready to go.

My moment came when Celtic were away at Hibs, at Easter Road, at the beginning of May. Martin had put me on the bench. At half-time, Martin turned round to me and said, 'Right Stubbsy, get your stuff ready, you are going on.' I went along the touchline to warm up, and as I was doing so, I could hear people clapping. The Celtic fans were cheering me and shouting my name, over and over. It caught me completely off guard.

I went over to the fourth official, ready to come on. Martin and Wally were with me.

'Go on and enjoy yourself,' Wally said.

'It's great to have you back,' Martin said. 'You deserve this.'

The fourth official held up my number, and the next thing I knew, the whole crowd were standing and applauding: the Hibs fans, the Celtic fans, all four sides of the ground were giving me an ovation. The Celtic fans were singing my name again and again. I had a lump in my throat, and could feel myself welling up. I had to fight back the tears. It was an incredible reaction, and a moment that will stay with me for the rest of my life.

I ran on to the pitch and didn't know what to do with myself. Suddenly I was back in the thick of it, running around and trying to get hold of the ball. Every time I touched it, the fans cheered. As the half went on, I started to have a bit of contact: the Hibs players were going for the ball and there'd be the usual pushing and pulling going on. As they pulled on me, I could feel my stomach: it was almost as if it was ripping. This isn't right, I thought to myself. This is all way too early. But there was no way I wasn't going to play. As far as I was concerned the ripping was just telling me that the wound had not completely healed as yet: it might have done on the outside, but the inner wall of the muscle wasn't quite a hundred per cent.

I couldn't get away from the ripping. Every time I jumped, or turned, or twisted, there it was. Nobody was going easy on me, and I wouldn't have expected them to. As far as they were concerned, if I was back on the pitch, then there were no favours granted. They were there to win the game. I was lifted in the air, felt the weight of some meaty tackles. I was given a proper workout that afternoon, no doubt about it. But I was so pleased to be back playing, I didn't care. To top off an amazing afternoon, I even got on the scoresheet: scoring Celtic's fourth goal in a 5–2 win.

The 2000–01 season was a fantastic one for Celtic. Martin's first season in charge saw us scoop a domestic treble, regaining the league title and winning both cups. For me, though, I'd won more: the team had won the treble, but in beating cancer I felt as though I'd won the quadruple. For all my achievements on the football pitch, I think that getting back on the pitch and playing again was the greatest one for me. I've played against some amazing opponents during my career, but cancer was the toughest one I've ever come up against. Played two, won two, against an opponent like cancer: it doesn't get much better than that.

Around the end of the season, I took a call from Paul Stretford, my agent at the time.

'I've been speaking to a club today who you would like to go to,' he said. 'A club in the North West.'

'Yeah right,' I said, jokingly. 'Who, Manchester United?'

'No, not them.'

'Manchester City?'

'No,' Paul said again.

'Blackburn?'

'Come on Alan, think about it.'

It was then that the penny dropped.

'Not . . . Everton?'

'I thought you'd never get there,' Paul laughed.

My heart skipped a beat. 'You are joking, aren't you? Is this some sort of wind-up?'

'I've been with them all afternoon,' Paul continued.

'And?' I asked, trying not to sound too excited. 'What did they say?'

'They want you to come down and meet them.'

To say this was the most difficult decision of my career was the understatement of the century. I loved Celtic. I'd had a fantastic five years there and they had been brilliant to me: the way the club had helped me through the cancer was a tribute to their class. They couldn't have done more for me, they really couldn't. Glasgow, too, was a great place to live. Mandy and I were extremely settled: in fact, we were probably the most settled we'd been since we moved up there. The children were happy at their school and we all loved living there. I would quite happily move back to Glasgow, to Scotland, tomorrow: I enjoyed it that much. At the same time, however, Everton was my club. It was my boyhood dream to one day pull on that blue shirt and hear the terraces of Goodison shouting my name.

I went to speak to Martin about it. Although my contract was up, I wanted to be upfront about the situation; after everything he'd done for me, it was the least I could do. Martin, once again, was fantastic about my dilemma. He knew Everton was my boyhood team, and understood exactly where I was coming from.

'Go down and speak to them,' he told me. 'But remember that if it's not quite right or it doesn't work out, your contract is still on the table. I still want you to sign for us.'

I was grateful for that, and for his generosity. I was completely torn, and Martin could see that. Part of me felt obliged to stay with Celtic: I owed them for what they'd done for me. And I think if it had been any other club in the world at that point, then I wouldn't have even gone to speak to them. But I couldn't turn down the chance of playing for Everton – a footballer's career is not a long one, and after the cancer, I was conscious of taking chances when they arose.

I drove down and had a meeting with Walter Smith, the Everton manager at the time. I met him at his house in Wilmslow, Manchester. It was just him, me and my agent, Paul. Walter had been manager of Rangers when I'd first gone up to Glasgow, so he knew a bit about me. We chatted about Everton and his plans for the team. Walter explained that the defender Richard Gough was leaving, and he was looking for someone to replace him. He explained how he was trying to do something at Everton, and wanted to make it a real success. He was quite honest, Walter: he explained that he didn't have a lot of money to spend on transfers, so was looking to bring in some quality free transfers to help with the budget. I ticked all the boxes as the sort of player he was looking for.

Walter told me to go away and think about it, but I knew immediately that I'd be signing. I went back to see Martin and told him that I wanted to go.

'I don't want to leave on bad terms,' I said. 'After everything the club has done for me . . .'

'Not at all,' Martin said. 'After all you have been through, you deserve this opportunity. It's your boyhood team and I fully understand. There's no hard feelings from me whatsoever.'

It is a dream of mine that if I do go into football management, then one day I get the chance to manage Celtic. Not because it is a big club or anything like that, but because I feel as though I have an awful lot to repay them for. I would love to go back, manage them and win the league for them. I think that would be hugely satisfying and a way of saying thank you to the club and fans for all the help and support they gave me through those difficult times.

I've been back to Celtic Park many times since I left. I played in a testimonial and got a great response from the fans when I went on the pitch – it was a wonderful welcome back and the feeling was mutual. I go back and watch games, both for pleasure and for professional reasons – Celtic always have some good players and Everton, like any club, keep tabs on that. I always enjoy going. I've played for some great clubs and Celtic was one it was a real privilege to play for. It is a special club.

I was excited about going to Everton, but publicly I kept a lid on it. I didn't want to be disrespectful to Celtic and avoided going to the papers and giving them one of those exclusives about how you're excited and thrilled at the challenge, even though I was. The truth was that I was both happy to be going to Everton and back to Liverpool, but also sad to be saying goodbye to Celtic and Scotland. I was leaving Celtic, but when you've spent that long at such an amazing club, in a way I wasn't. If you've played for Celtic, it never really leaves you, and certainly, it has never left me.

# 12

## Goodison, Gazza and Grav

There was only one person who was more pleased than me to be signing for Everton: my dad. As soon as I knew I was signing, I couldn't wait to tell him. He didn't know I'd been down to see Walter Smith, so when I went to tell him the news, it was a complete surprise.

'Dad,' I said on the phone, trying to sound casual. 'I'm going to be popping in for a minute. I've got something to tell you.'

It wasn't until I got there that I told him. 'Oh, and by the way, I'm signing for Everton tomorrow.'

You should have seen his face. 'You're joking,' he said.

'Straight up,' I replied.

Then he came straight over and gave me this massive hug. He was chuffed to bits.

Throughout my time at Celtic, it was my dad who kept me in touch with what was going on at Everton. He read the *Echo* every night, and would fill me in with all the gossip. He always wanted me to play for Everton and wasn't shy in telling people, 'Our Alan should be at Everton'. I was pleased for him that he could see me play for them: that moment when I walked out at Goodison for the first time as an Everton player, he'd have been as proud as anything. I was glad that I managed to provide him with that feeling.

I was glad, too, that I could help him out with tickets and the like. He'd never been a season ticket holder, because he couldn't afford it: he'd always been a 'transistor to the ear' sort of a fan. Now I was playing for Everton, I could get him tickets and passes into the players' lounge. He was like a child in a sweet shop, and would always be going up to Big Dunc and the other players and asking for a photograph.

'Dad!' I'd wind him up. 'You're in your sixties, you're not some kid, you know!'

My playing for Everton meant a lot to him: it meant a lot to me as well. Throughout my career, I'd always had that winning mentality. Once I was on the pitch, I just wanted to win. But playing for Everton, winning somehow mattered to me that little bit more. I was playing for the fans, I was playing for myself as an Evertonian. I was playing for all my family and friends who were Everton fans. There was an added pressure to win as I didn't want to spend my Saturday evening explaining to them why we'd lost!

The moment for me when it all hit home was walking out for the first time. I remember walking down the tunnel from the dressing room, and hearing the theme tune of *Z-Cars* being piped out over the tannoy. There's a placard on the wall as you go out, right above your head: Home of the Blues, it says. When I was a boy, I'd been on a tour of Goodison and had touched this sign. One day, I'd thought to myself, I'll do that as a player. As I went out onto the pitch that first time, I touched the sign with my hand, an Everton player. I felt invigorated. I've made it, I thought. I'm here at last.

It was strange to think how I'd gone full circle – starting out as an Everton boy and now here, towards the end of my career, I was back and playing for the team. I was back at Bellefield, the training ground where I'd done all my sessions as a boy. That was a bit of a nostalgia kick. Once I'd been the boy hanging around the gates with an autograph book, hoping to catch Reidy or Graeme Sharp on their way out. Now there were boys of the same age hanging about and asking for my autograph.

The coach at the academy who'd let me go, he was no longer part of the set-up. But he lived locally and I'd see him around: there were no hard feelings from me about his decision whatsoever. I wasn't the first footballer to be released who went on to make it elsewhere. It's something that Everton themselves have done on more than one occasion – they did the same thing to Phil Jagielka and Leighton Baines. Those are two big examples of where the wrong call was made, but in each case thankfully the players came back. And in terms of the decision making at the Academy, they are the exceptions. Everton have a good reputation for producing young players for a reason.

It's fair to say that when I joined Everton, the team had been enjoying a topsy-turvy few years. The championship winning success of Howard Kendall's eighties team that I had watched growing up felt a long time past. The club had won the FA Cup under Joe Royle in 1995 but that had been the only recent bit of silverware to fill the trophy cupboard. Howard Kendall had been brought back as a manager for another stint, and for whatever reason, the original spark that made him such a success wasn't there. Mike Walker had come in, and that hadn't worked out either, and it was at that point that the club had turned to Walter Smith.

There was also plenty going on behind the scenes that hadn't helped matters. There had been the whole Peter Johnson episode, the debacle of his attempts to take over the club and then his leaving. There was an incident when Duncan Ferguson was sold behind the manager's back, which hadn't gone down well with anyone – the manager, the players, the fans, Big Dunc himself. It wasn't until the new chairman, Bill Kenwright, had come in, that Duncan returned to the team.

Bill is still chairman today. He has come in for a bit of criticism from the fans, who have felt frustrated by the attempts to grow the club. I think that's unfair – Bill has been there and provided first Walter, and then David Moyes, with everything he can. He's gone to every length to try and bring in new investment. One of the criticisms that some fans make is that he hasn't tried to actively sell the club. The thing is, though, that Bill is a fan of the club. He doesn't just want to sell it to any Tom, Dick or Harry to make a bit of money. For every successful story of an investor buying a Premier League team, there are plenty of other ones where the buyer hasn't delivered the goods. Bill is a different character to Fergus McCann but they are similar in one way – like Fergus, Bill wants to leave his club in a good state, and passed over to someone they feel are a safe pair of hands.

Although Celtic and Everton are different, there are similarities between the two clubs. The set-up of the clubs in terms of people they employ is quite similar – the only thing that differs is the size of each department. David Moyes famously described Everton as 'the people's club' and I think the same could be said about Celtic in Scotland as well. Certainly, there is a difference in the make-up of fan bases of Everton and Liverpool. Because of the latter's European success, their audience has always been more global than Everton's. Through the seventies and eighties, Liverpool would have a lot of young children and teenagers who supported Liverpool, even though they were not from the area. The same is true of Manchester United in the nineties and noughties.

In comparison to Liverpool, Everton has had to rely more on their fans from the city, simply because we have not been so successful. That was what David Moyes was driving at when he described Everton as the people's club. You look at Goodison on a match day, and the make-up of the crowd is predominantly from the city: you get more people from Liverpool at Everton than you do at Anfield. That's not a slight on Liverpool: some people tried to spin a negative slant on what Moyesey said, but I never thought that was his intention. It was an honest statement as to where he thought the club was at.

The closeness of the relationship between Everton and the local community was brought into focus a few years later, with the tragic death of Rhys Jones. Rhys had been no different to me: he was a typical local lad, grew up in a working class suburb of Liverpool, was football mad and an Everton fan. Rhys had been cycling home after playing football when he had been shot dead. It was a senseless killing, an absolute tragedy, shocking the city to its core. Everton as a club immediately got in touch with the family and asked if we could help in any way. The squad went down to the pub carpark in Croxteth Park where he had been killed, and laid a wreath, to show our support.

When it came to Rhys's funeral, the family asked the club to be involved. I was asked as a local lad if I would give the reading and it was the absolute least I could do. The funeral took place at Liverpool Cathedral, and it was one of those events that brought the whole community together. I'll never forget seeing that tiny coffin, blue and white with an Everton crest on it. I was petrified about giving the reading: I was nervous about speaking, but more that I wanted to do right for Rhys's family. I managed to get through it okay, thankfully, and was very proud to have been able to do that for them.

*　　*　　*

When I first joined Everton, they had not really being doing as well as a club their size should have been. The team had been down at the wrong end of the table and relegation had been a real possibility. We hadn't gone down, however, and that's because there were strong characters in that dressing room, both on the pitch and off it.

It was funny having played against Gazza so many times up in Scotland to now find myself on the same team as him. Gazza was coming to the end of his career by the time he joined Everton. He still had his magic, but it wasn't for the full ninety minutes by this point – but every so often you'd see a flash in a match or on the training ground, and you'd be reminded of what an amazing player he was. He was a great person to have around the dressing room, funny and warm, and everyone loved him.

Walter knew Gazza well from their time together up in Scotland, and knew how to handle him. He was almost like a father figure to him at times. Walter was aware of what Gazza got up to off the pitch, and there were times where he would take him in, and have Gazza stay with him. Gazza didn't get shouted at in the same way as the other players: that wasn't the way to get the best out of him. He was fragile, and at times frustrated at getting older. His mind still knew what he wanted to do on the pitch, but his body couldn't always deliver. You could see signs of him starting to fall away as a player, and it was painful to watch because he had such a height to fall from. It was painful to watch, too, because I knew it would happen to me one day as well.

Gazza's footballing gifts might have diminished, but his mischievous sense of humour remained as strong as ever. When I first moved back to Liverpool, I was staying in the same hotel as Gazza for a time. One incident between Gazza and his friend,

Jimmy 'Five Bellies' Gardner, stands out. Jimmy wanted to take his family on holiday and had asked Gazza for some money. Gazza wouldn't give him any money until Jimmy had 'done something' for him. Usually this would involve driving him somewhere, or going to pick something up for him. On this occasion, Gazza was bored and wanted Jimmy to do something daft. There was a teaspoon on the table, and Gazza picked it up, lit his lighter and starting burning the spoon.

'No Gazza,' Jimmy said, instantly. 'I'm not doing that. Whatever it is you're about to suggest, I'm not going to do it.'

'All right,' said Gazza, continuing to hold the flame against the spoon. 'Then I'm not going to give you any money for your holiday.'

'Ah, come on,' Jimmy pleaded. 'I promised my family I'd take them away.'

Gazza was still holding the lighter against the spoon. By now it was getting red hot.

'Put this on the end of your nose,' Gazza said. 'Spoon on your nose and you can have your money.'

'Gazza, I can't. No. Fuck off, no way. I'm not doing that.'

'Then you're not getting your money.' Gazza held the spoon out to him. 'This is your last chance.'

Jimmy was shaking his head, saying 'Oh fuck, Gazza, oh shit.' He really didn't want to do it, but he wanted the money. He took the spoon and held it close to his nose. Close enough that he could feel the heat coming off it.

'I can't do it,' he said, and put the spoon down on the table.

'Do it,' Gazza said, 'or you are not going to get your money.'

'But it's going to burn my nose . . .'

On this went, and all the time the spoon was beginning to cool down a little. Gazza spotted this, and flicked his lighter on again. 'I'm going to have to heat it up again.'

At this, Jimmy snatched the spoon up again, put it up right to his nose, wavering. 'I can't do this, I can't do this . . .' he muttered. And then the next minute, he *did* do it. He banged the spoon onto his nose and all you could hear was this *'Sssss . . .'* sound. Jimmy pulls it away, and in doing so, takes the skin off his nose. He's in agony, just saying, 'Fucking hell, Gazza' again and again, and Gazza is on the floor in stitches, laughing his head off.

'I can't believe you actually did it,' he said.

Jimmy's nose comes right up, there's this huge bubble blister on it. I think he ended up having to go to hospital to get it sorted out. But he got his holiday. And that was Gazza all over.

Another famous name we had at the club at the time was David Ginola. His signing was a bit of a gamble: David was another flair player and had been a fan's favourite at Newcastle and Tottenham. Like Gazza, he was a player getting towards the end of his career and although you saw it at times, he lacked the sparkle of old. When he joined the club, Gazza welcomed him in the only way he knew how: he came out for that training session wearing this long black wig, in imitation of David's famous flowing locks. He was stroking his hair and flicking it backwards like he was in a shampoo advert. Everyone thought this was hilarious, with the possible exception of David. He never really settled at the club and only played half a dozen games.

Up front, the club's talisman was Duncan Ferguson – Big Dunc. He was a pivotal figure, both in the dressing room and on the pitch. The fans loved him. I thought he was a top drawer footballer. He didn't always get the accolades that his talent deserved, but he was a great player. I saw how good he was, day in day out, on the training pitch, and had the bruises to show for it! Dunc was fantastic in the air, and was very, very good on the floor. He had great feet: he could score with either foot, but he could make goals as well. He was a good fit for Everton. The way the team was set-up allowed him to play his game, probably more so than any other team he played for. It was just a shame that he had a couple of niggly injuries at the time, which meant that he didn't play as much as he'd have liked to.

Dunc was the sort of player you wanted on your team. Part of the reason why the fans loved him was that even when he wasn't playing well, you knew he'd still put his heart and soul into it, and would fight for Everton no matter what. Off the pitch, he was quiet, and quite reserved. He was a family man at heart and I got on well with him: we'd go out and socialise together. I was always touched by that, because I knew that Dunc didn't let that many people in. He had a close circle of friends and that was it. If you were lucky enough to spend time with him, he was fantastic company. Very loyal, too, the sort of person you could talk to, confident it would go no further; the sort of friend who would have your back and support you one hundred and ten per cent.

Another key player when I joined was David Weir, who was to be my partner in the centre of defence. Davy and I immediately formed an understanding and developed what was one of the strongest pairings of my career. Neither of us was the quickest, but we made up for that with our reading of the game and our support for each other. It probably helped that we defended deep, but we never let ourselves get exposed by pace: we knew how to put ourselves in the right place and avoid those situations. We were well balanced as a pair, and could play on the left or right. It meant that I always felt confident that if I was dragged out of position, Davy would be there to cover.

Later on in my Everton career, I was paired up with Joseph Yobo: he was a great player in his own way, but we never had the same sort of understanding. Joseph was athletic and a very power-ful player: he was quick, strong in the air and fantastic in a one vs one situation. But he was also more interested in himself: if I was dragged out of position, I knew that Davy would have my back; I was never sure whether or not Joseph would come across and help me.

Thomas Gravesen in midfield was another very gifted player, and an absolute oddball to boot. He had this crazy streak to him. Gazza was a practical joker, but his jokes were always done in jest. Thomas's messing around had more of an edge, I felt. He'd grab people in headlocks and mess about with them on the treatment tables. He'd bring paintball guns with him to training and would fire them at you. When Bonfire Night came round, he'd buy a load of fireworks and bring them in and set them off.

Then there were his wheels. The parking lot at the training ground was stuffed with flash cars; Thomas, though, would turn up in a Nissan Micra. 'Look at that,' he'd say to our bemused looks, 'what a car'. The next week he'd turn up in a Porsche Turbo. That's what I mean about him: completely nuts, and completely unpredictable. This side of his character made its way onto the pitch as well. He was phenomenally gifted as a footballer, but a nightmare for the manager from the discipline point of view – he'd do something ridiculous with the ball, but then disappear off out of position and leave you exposed. He went on to play for Real Madrid, but still kept his apartment in Liverpool.

Tomasz Radzinski signed for Everton around the same time that I did. He was a little fizz bomb of a striker and had real pace. He was so fast, in fact, that it could almost be a hindrance to him. He'd get himself in position so quick that he could not set himself for the finish. He made a great start for Everton and scored a few goals, but eventually only stayed for a couple of seasons before moving on. To be fair, we have had a lot of strikers at Everton in my time: that is the one area where the managers have gone through more players than any other.

Walter's right-hand man on the training ground was Archie Knox. Archie took most of the training and did the day to day coaching: Walter would sit back, watch and observe. Archie was the loud one, the shouter and screamer. He was from the 'fucking this' and 'fucking that' school of coaching. Walter, by contrast, was the quiet, calm one. Well, until he lost his rag anyway. When he let rip, he really let rip. Cups would be thrown, skips booted if he didn't like what he saw on the pitch. The players were under no illusions as to what it was he meant and wanted out of you.

Out of all the managers I've played for, Walter was one of the most powerful when it came to losing it. Bruce Rioch was fierce, but it was always there with him, close to the surface: he'd go through you on the training ground without a second thought. Walter was more reserved. It took a lot more to make him explode, but when he did, he more than made up for lost time.

The players would take this from Walter, but not so much from Archie. I was a seasoned professional by this point, and like the other older heads in the dressing room, someone shouting at you is not always the best way to get you motivated. There's an element of having seen it all before of getting the hairdryer treatment. Sometimes, the shouting can be counter-productive: rather than firing someone up, they can end up taking offence. That happened on a number of occasions with Archie: he'd had a go at someone, they hadn't liked it, and the next thing you knew they were almost coming to blows.

It's not the end of the world when that happens. It's good that emotions are running high: it shows they're passionate about the club and wanting to do well. If you've got a coach who knows his job is on the line, and a player who won't accept they're in the wrong, then there's always going to be a flashpoint. That's the dressing room, for you. There's nowhere to hide.

Those arguments continued throughout my opening season at Everton. We got off to an absolute flier: after three or four matches we were top of the league. But from there, the results began to slide and by spring, the team were once more heading back down towards the wrong end of the table. We weren't quite there yet, but it was one of those situations where the team could find themselves dragged into another relegation battle.

There started to be murmurings about Walter's job being on the line. I remember we were playing Stoke in the FA Cup and word went round that if we lost, then Walter would be sacked that evening. Whether those rumours were true or not, we went out and I scored the winner that day. I was pleased to do that, not just to win the match, but for Walter as well. The players were behind Walter and wanted to do well for him. But as hard as we tried for him, the results just didn't come and after another disappointing result against Middlesbrough, the chairman decided it was time for him to go.

One of the things that has been noticeable since I've been at Everton is what a good relationship the chairman has always had with the manager. Even ending Walter's reign, Bill called him in for a chat and they agreed that it wasn't working out. It says something that Bill and Walter are still good friends: their relationship survived the business decision that the chairman had to make. It's no coincidence that the same thing has happened between Bill and David Moyes as well: their relationship has grown over the years, and has helped both of them.

David was Walter's replacement. He was young – only thirty-eight – but had done fantastically well up the road with Preston, and Bill decided he was ready to manage at the top level. David was someone who had done his time at Celtic as a boy and teenager, but had taken an interest in coaching from a young age. In fact, he took his coaching badges early on in his playing-career.

At Preston, he'd put together an attractive young team: he had pushed them and dragged them up. David was clearly ambitious, and had that fear factor over the young players. He was firm, had an edge to him and the players knew what was expected of them.

When you've got a young team, you can push them to work hard and can say things to them because of their age. When David first came to Everton, he tried to carry on that management style. He quickly found out how strong the personalities were in the dressing room, and that he wouldn't be able to treat us or speak to us in the same way as with the Preston players. At Preston, David could have fined a player a week's wages – that's a big deal when you're not on a huge amount of money and so they'd do what he said to avoid it. At Everton, where the players were earning Premier League salaries, the response to such a fine was simply, so what?

This was all new to him. I don't think David had experienced players standing up and telling him what they thought: he probably didn't have so many at Preston who would question his authority. David was smart about it, though. The easiest thing to do would have been to say, 'This is my way, and if you don't like it, you can go.' That, though, would have been bad management. Particularly given the situation Everton were in, he needed the better players on his side from the start.

You don't have long as a manager to get the respect of the players. If you've played professionally, then the players will give you a certain degree of respect to start with, because they know you've been there and done it. That, though, only lasts a short period of time: as John Barnes found at Celtic. If you haven't been a player, someone like Andre Villas-Boas for example, then you've got to prove yourself from the start. When AVB took over at Chelsea, he found seasoned and experienced international players thinking,

'Who are you to tell me what to do when you have never kicked a ball in your life?' Whatever your previous footballing experience, a new manager doesn't have long to get it right: the players can sniff out whether or not someone knows what they are talking about, and whether they can put those words into practice on the training ground.

That was what David was brilliant at. Right from the word go, he was in control on the training ground. He was very clear in getting his message across – what he wanted from us, and how he wanted us to play. David explained how he was ambitious and knew exactly where he wanted to go. But right at that point, given the situation Everton were in, it was all about results. Get those, keep Everton safe, and then the club could think bigger about the following season. David was rigorous in assessing each of us as players, and the teams he chose were the ones he thought would achieve instant results.

Tactically, David was big on defence. He wanted his defenders to defend and didn't want us taking risks. You get a strong defensive platform, and you give the team the best possible chance of winning. That was our job as a back four: to keep a clean sheet and not give any set-pieces away. I wasn't totally happy about it at the time: there were moments when I thought to myself, I'm 31 years old and I'm doing header practice? I wasn't the only one either. But looking back, David was right to drill us like that. He wanted us to think about our positions on the pitch, so that if a ball came in from whatever angle, we'd know exactly where it was we were meant to be. If one of the defenders went for the ball, where should the other three be if he misses the header? It was that sort of thing.

I had a moan about it at the start, but as we went on, I realised that it gave me a sense of confidence: I'd be on the pitch and know exactly where I was meant to be. I knew my job and sometimes that simplicity of task can help a team. Certainly, the team got an immediate uplift after David's appointment. In his first match in charge against Fulham, David Unsworth scored after just thirty seconds. We went on to win the match and that set the tone for the rest of the season. We survived the drop with something to spare.

# 13

---

# Wonderboy Wayne

Right from the start of my time at Everton, there was talk about this prodigiously talented young player coming through the ranks: this fourteen, fifteen-year-old who was playing for the Under-16s, Under-17s and youth team. His name, of course, was Wayne Rooney. The fact that Wayne was a local lad only added to the buzz about him inside the club. I remember going to watch him in some of the youth games and being blown away by what I saw. There was an FA Youth Cup tournament where he nearly won it single-handedly for us. In the final against Aston Villa, Wayne was away with England for the first leg and we got beaten 3–1. In the return leg, when he was back, we drew. Had he been available for both legs, I'm sure we would have won. That's how influential he already was.

Watching him play for the youth team, it was difficult sometimes to tell who was the fifteen-year-old kid, and who were the seventeen and eighteen-year-olds. Quite simply, he was by far the most gifted player I had ever seen for that age. He had touch, vision, movement and a football brain beyond his years. Wayne had football strength, by which I mean he knew how to use his body: something that players don't normally get until they are far more experienced. Things like being able to push himself off the defender to gain an extra couple of yards: that requires both understanding and strength to achieve, especially at that age when your opponent is older than you are.

There was pressure for Walter to bring him up to train with the first team. Even though Walter knew all about Wayne, he was resistant to begin with, to throw someone that young into the limelight and that level of intensity. But towards the end of his reign, he relented and Wayne came up to train with us. As a pro, you get this fifteen-year-old coming up to join you, and there's an element of wanting to put this kid in his place. But it was difficult to dislike Wayne: he was quite quiet, and clearly excited to be there. The thing about Wayne is that nothing fazes him. The only thing that seemed to make him pause was Big Dunc; Wayne was a proper Evertonian and Big Dunc was his hero: you could see he was in awe of the guy.

It's funny to think that for a couple of months, there was this overlap at the club between Wayne and Gazza: the greatest player of one generation coming to the end of his career, and the greatest player of another just beginning his. I don't know whether they talked – Gazza was a bit in and out by the end, but he would have seen how talented Wayne was, and it would be nice to think he passed something on. One difference between the two of them was their family support. Gazza had a difficult childhood, which has probably not helped him later on in life; Wayne, by contrast, came from a strong and solid family background. He was always well grounded from the start.

I got to know Wayne well, almost immediately. We were both local lads and Evertonians and hit it off. I used to give him a lift to training as he was too young to drive, and would try to answer any questions he had about the game. I encouraged that: I remember how important the senior players had been when I first started, and told Wayne that any problems he had, he should just give me a shout. I think he appreciated that. We became good friends and remained so, even after he moved to United.

David Moyes was good for Wayne. I think he looked at how Sir Alex Ferguson had dealt with his generation of young players – Beckham, Scholes, Giggs and so on – and tried to keep Wayne out of the limelight. He kept him away from doing any sort of media stuff, and attempted to protect him as much as he could. That's difficult when the player has a rise like Wayne did. In the following pre-season, Wayne scored nine goals; he became the club's youngest scorer in a Worthington Cup match against Wrexham. The clamour from Everton fans for him to start grew and grew, but David used him sparingly, bringing him on as a substitute.

The game when Wayne really announced his arrival to the world was when Arsenal came to Goodison in October 2002. I was on the bench that day, alongside Wayne. Arsenal were the league champions at the time and came to Merseyside on a thirty-odd match unbeaten run. They were a fantastic side, with David Seaman in goal, Sol Campbell and Ashley Cole at the back, Vieira and Ljungberg in midfield and Thierry Henry up front. It was no surprise, then, when Arsenal went in front, Freddie Ljungberg scoring after just seven minutes. But we struck back, with Tomasz Radzinski levelling the scores halfway through the first half.

It was a good game of football with plenty of chances at both ends as the match wore on. Wayne came on with ten minutes to go to huge cheers from the crowd. Then, as full-time neared and the game still all square, Thomas Gravesen found Wayne with a looping pass. Wayne watched the ball come down and took it on his instep. He twisted away from the defenders marking him and walloped a shot from 25 yards out. It crashed in off the inside of the crossbar, beating David Seaman all ends up. As debut league goals went, it was right up there.

It was no surprise to anyone at the club. When Wayne was picked for England and went on to make his name at Euro 2004 in Portugal, it again seemed the natural trajectory of his talent. It was fantastic to have him on your side: he was just fearless. When you are that young, you have this freedom from playing without pressure; you don't care who you are playing against, you just want to play. I think David Moyes worked out quite quickly that he didn't have to tell Wayne what to do. When people are that talented, they work it out for themselves. Everton didn't need to coach Wayne – he was good enough that he coached himself. We were just there to help him with his development.

It soon dawned on the players that we were not going to have Wayne around for long. It seemed inevitable that he would go elsewhere. The big clubs were hovering, and there were scouts coming down to watch every game. Wayne knew this, and we chatted about it: Manchester United, Arsenal and Real Madrid were just some of the teams who were sending people across to check him out. Particularly after the Euros, it didn't seem a question of when Wayne would go, but at what price.

Wayne asked me what I thought and I was quite straight with him. Of course, part of me wanted him to stay at Everton: the part of me that was an Everton fan certainly didn't want him to go. But it made sense for him to leave in terms of his career. I told him that I thought Real Madrid, though exciting, wouldn't have been quite right for him – I felt he was too young to go abroad and thrive. Out of the English clubs, Manchester United always felt the right fit for him. He would still be close to home, and would benefit from playing for one of the best managers that the game had ever seen. Sir Alex would be the father figure who would be able to help his development. I told Wayne that if I was him, that was where I'd go.

The fans weren't happy when Wayne left, of course not. I think the situation was heightened because Wayne wasn't just a great footballer, but because he was a local lad and Everton fan as well. He was one of us. Some fans felt that he went too early and could have stayed a couple more seasons. He could have done, but you never know what might have been around the corner. He could have stayed and had a cruciate injury or broken his leg. At that point, the opportunity would have gone. As it was, the club got £27 million for him, which was a fantastic amount of money.

Some fans suggested that because Wayne and I shared the same agent – Paul Stretford – that was why I gave Wayne the advice about moving to Manchester United. That wasn't true. Paul never asked me to give Wayne any advice or steer. In fact, at the time my relationship with Paul wasn't great: we'd had a bit of a falling out because I hadn't gone to his wedding as I had a family holiday already booked. With Wayne, I didn't help him move to Manchester United. I just told him as a friend what I felt would be best for him.

I'll tell you one thing I'm fairly sure about though. I think Wayne will come back and play for Everton again one day. Wayne might be a United player, but he remains an Everton fan. There would be nothing better than to see Wayne return to the club, pull on that blue shirt again and play at Goodison at the end of his career. You only have to look at Kai, his son. What was Kai's first football kit? An Everton one. That, for me, tells you everything.

The results in the first few seasons of David's reign couldn't have been more different. The season he took over from Walter, we ended up finishing fifteenth; in David's first full season in charge, we finished seventh; the following season we were seventeenth; the next we finished fourth.

It's difficult to give a reason as to why that was so: on a longer view, the club had been a little bit 'yo-yo' for a while. It takes time for any squad to get used to a new manager; there's always a period of transition where the team gets changed, and the former manager's players go and the new transfers come in. So maybe that might have had something to do with it. The season we finished seventeenth was Wayne's last, but I wouldn't put any blame on the uncertainty and rumour as to whether or not he would stay. Anytime someone uses that sort of thing as an excuse, I always think it's a bit of a cop out. The players are the professionals on the pitch: you should do your job and leave the media professionals to do their job off it.

There has been this habit with Everton for sometimes being something of a slow starter as a team. I couldn't tell you why, but there have been a number of seasons where we haven't started the season particularly well, and only found our gear after Christmas. Sometimes, the fixture computer can give you a tricky start to the season, you begin at the wrong end of the table and never find your momentum. Before you know it, you find yourself flirting around the relegation places and the season becomes a battle for survival.

That's what happened in 2003–04. We only won three of our first fifteen games, and two of those were against clubs who would go on to be relegated. December saw an improvement, and we enjoyed wins against Portsmouth, Leicester and Birmingham, and for a while it looked as though we'd kick on to safety. As it was, our next victory didn't come until the end of February. Even after that, we only won two out of our last eleven games, and lost our last four. We ended up with 39 points, which in many years would have got us relegated, but we knew before the last day of the season that we were safe. A bad season ended on a bad note with a dead rubber against Manchester City, who had also only just avoided relegation. They celebrated by thumping us 5–1. It was a terrible way to finish things, and sad that it was Wayne's last game in an Everton shirt.

The team felt humiliated to have finished seventeenth. No player ever wants to be involved in relegation. It is not a nice way to play football. You find yourself playing under pressure: there's hostility from the fans and added bite to the opposition, who sense blood. Once you're down there, that's when players end up doing things they would not normally do on the pitch. It's nothing to do with the quality of the players: it's all about anxiety, nervousness, and being aware of what the consequences are. All of that affects your decision making. Some players simply cope better with the pressure than others. Others just crumble. What probably kept us up that season was the fact that we had a strong group of players – experienced characters who could dig deep when it counted. We knew we had the quality, as this was basically the same squad that had finished seventh the season before. The positive, if there was one, to take from the season was the confirmation that we had the character to match.

I don't know what odds you'd have got on Everton getting into the Champions League places the following season. Certainly, the pundits had us tipped for relegation, a belief seemingly confirmed by the sale of Wayne to Manchester United and a bad opening day of the season: a 4–1 defeat to Arsenal at Goodison, with Dennis Bergkamp having a blinder. Our next game took us away to Crystal Palace, and to the delight of the home fans we were one-down within ten minutes.

Then, though, things started to change. Palace should have made it two-nil, but I managed to clear the ball off the line and keep us in the game. We got a penalty before half-time, which Grav put away, and were right back in it. Tommy scored again in the second half and made another: we ended up winning 3–1, the first time we had won away from home for nine months, and our season was up and running.

Although Wayne had gone, David had brought in some quality players over the summer: Tim Cahill had arrived from Millwall and Marcus Bent had been brought in from Ipswich. Later on in the season, the squad would be augmented by James Beattie and Mikel Arteta, who arrived on loan from Real Sociedad. Going forward, then, we had a lot of options, while at the back we had the solid experience on which to build from. It was a nice balance.

There was to be no slow Everton start that season: we kicked on and after beating Palace, won five of our next six games: the only one we didn't was a draw at Old Trafford. Far from thinking about the drop zone, we were enjoying life at the top of the table, and keeping pace with the early leaders: we spent Christmas in third place, behind only Chelsea and Arsenal.

On top of which, that December was the first time I'd played in a Liverpool derby and ended up on the winning side. In fact, throughout my time playing at Everton, although there were countless draws I think we only ever beat Liverpool twice. To beat our local rivals was what every Everton fan wanted more than anything, but to do so was a massive challenge. Liverpool were consistently getting into the Champions League at the time and had a squad to reflect that: they were getting twenty million plus a year from competing in Europe, whereas Everton might have only got five or six million to improve the squad. When you look at it like that, then Liverpool should have been beating us.

None of that took away from the fact that as an Evertonian myself, being beaten by them was absolutely the worst feeling. More than any other game in the season, the derbies were the ones I was desperate to win. I would have run through a brick wall, drawn blood, anything, to walk out of Goodison or Anfield with a victory over Liverpool.

The derbies were the games in the season where you had to work hard not to let your emotions take over. I couldn't have been more aware of how much we were carrying the expectations of the fans on our shoulders. For the local lads like myself, Leon Osman and Tony Hibbert, it meant everything, and we'd try and get that across to the other players. Such emotion can be a difficult thing to handle in this situation. It's possible to lose a game in the dressing room before the match: everyone can get so worked up that by the time you get onto the pitch, it all feels a little flat. Sometimes, you can find yourself playing as though all the nervous tension has been sucked out of you. That can be half the battle at times, just to get on the pitch in the right frame of mind.

Quite often in those derbies, Liverpool just seemed to cope with the occasion better than we did. Their big players were always in the right frame of mind to produce on the day, and no one did that more so than Steven Gerrard. He was their talisman, and there were derby matches where he was single-handedly the reason that Liverpool won. He was a top, top player to play against. I admire him alot as a player and what he has achieved for his club.

That said, it didn't stop me hating him or his team-mates for the ninety minutes I was against them on the pitch. That was the way I was. I wanted to win for Everton and the team, and I automatically didn't like anyone on the other side. With Liverpool, it was more so. That was only ever for the duration of the match; I'd give it some banter and abuse during the game, and would expect to get some back, but once the final whistle went, I would shake their hand and it would all be forgotten.

There'd be a bit of edge to some of the banter – fuck you this and wanker that – and especially among the local lads: with Stevie and Jamie Carragher, especially. It could get a little personal, but as far as I was concerned, what was said on the pitch, was left there. Sometimes, however, people can take these comments a little too seriously. Jamie Carragher, who was a boyhood Evertonian before signing for Liverpool, wrote about me in his autobiography, and it's something that people sometimes mention. But you know what? I never even bothered to find out what he said about me. I know what I am on the pitch, and I am not the same as the guy off it: when I played, I played to win, not to be friends with someone.

There was one time after a derby match, I can't remember which one, and I went up to shake Jamie's hand. As I went to shake it, I ended up squeezing his hand really hard. It was one of those spontaneous things you do where as soon as you do it, you think, now why have I gone and done that? It was the emotion getting the better of me. Was it the right thing to do? I probably thought so at the time, but looking back it wasn't. Unless you are in that situation, though, it's difficult to know exactly what you would do.

I've been lucky as a player to have played in two of football's great derbies – Everton–Liverpool and Celtic–Rangers. It's interesting to compare how the rivalries matched up. One of the differences is that there was less socialising between the players in Merseyside than in Glasgow. Up in Scotland, the Celtic lads would come across the Rangers players, and we'd stop and have a drink. I think that probably used to be the case in Liverpool, too, perhaps ten or twenty years earlier. Now, however, a lot of their players live over the water: Heswall, Manchester, or wherever. Because they're going out in different places, our paths don't cross as much. There would be times when I was out in the same bar as Steven Gerrard, and he'd always offer to buy me a drink, or send one over, but those occasions were pretty rare.

Although the rivalry in Liverpool was fierce, it never had the sectarian edge of what I'd experienced in Glasgow. It was all quite tame by comparison – 'Everton scum! Stubbs, you're fucking shit!' – and I wore it like a badge of honour. If someone's shouting that sort of thing at you, it usually means you are doing all right. I probably got more grief out on the town in Liverpool than in Glasgow. There were plenty of Liverpool fans who would show you some respect: you're a really good player, they'd say, you're just playing for the wrong team. But there were others who'd give you a little comment as you went past: shout 'Blue twat' at you as they'd leg it round the corner to their mates. Sometimes, they'd give you a nudge on purpose so you'd turn round.

I normally just laugh. At the end of the day, I was a fan who loved playing for Everton. I never thought I'd do that in my lifetime, and always felt privileged and lucky to have played for the club. If someone wanted to walk past me, give me a nudge or call me a wanker because I played for Everton, then that would be their choice. But I knew that they would never be able to do what I had done: played for *my* team.

In the second half of the 2004–05 season, our form wasn't quite as good as at the start. We were probably disrupted a bit by the January sale of Gravesen to Real Madrid, but were good enough to keep ahead in a three-way fight for fourth with Liverpool and, of all teams, Bolton. We beat Newcastle 2–0 in early May, which, after Liverpool lost at Highbury the following day, was enough to secure us fourth place with two games to go.

We all met up on the Sunday in Liverpool and the manager took us for a night out and a bit of a celebration. We had a midweek game against Arsenal, and the Everton fans piled down to show their support. Unfortunately, it was one of those matches when everything went wrong. The Gaffer had made a few changes to the team – we'd qualified and he wanted to give a few of the other players a chance, so I found myself on the bench. Arsenal were on fire that night: one nil became two, became three by half-time. In the second half, it just got worse; four, five, six. I remember sitting on the bench next to Dunc and both of us were saying to each other, 'I really don't want to be going on to that'. Every time the Gaffer turned round, as though he might put us on, we slid down in our seats, in the hope he wouldn't see us! You should have seen Dunc's face when David told him to get ready. I stayed where I was, thank goodness, but the scoreline wasn't great – it finished 7–0 to Arsenal. I have joked about it with the Gaffer once or twice since, but no one was laughing that night. David made the players go and apologise to the fans at the end of the match.

It was a bittersweet moment, but although the result took the shine off things for 24 hours, it couldn't detract from what a fantastic achievement finishing fourth had been. I think that's particularly so, because the overall standard of the Premier League a decade ago was higher than it is today. This was a season where Liverpool, who went on to win the Champions League, could only finish fifth. I don't think that the Premier League today has the same depth to it than it did then: the top clubs are still strong, but lower down the division, there is not the gap to the Championship that there used to be. You can see that from how few clubs who came up used to stay up, and how much regularly the promoted teams survive now. The depth in the league isn't there in the same way. To qualify for the Champions League in the early noughties, you were doing so by regularly beating a lot of good teams.

There's this debate among fans sometimes about what is the bigger prize: to finish fourth in the league or win a trophy like the

FA Cup. I'm friends with Joe Parkinson, who was part of Everton's FA Cup winning team in 1995, and we joke about whose was the bigger achievement.

'Tell you what, Alan,' he teases, 'you can come and look at my medal any time.'

What have you got to show for finishing fourth? A printout of a league table on a piece of paper? Yet finishing fourth is the harder thing to do. To win the FA Cup, you only have to win six matches; to qualify for the Champions League, you have to do the business over thirty-eight games. I reckon it's one of those situations where the head says that fourth place is the bigger deal, but the heart says the trophy. Any player, like Joe, who has won the FA Cup will tell you they'd rather win that, and I think that would be the choice of most fans, too. Ask the board of directors, however, and from a financial point of view they'd rather be in the Champions League.

It probably depends a bit, too, on where the club is. For a club like Everton, we are not at a stage where we can look at ourselves as being contenders for the league. We have got our own 'league' to win, and finishing fourth is our equivalent. For a club like Arsenal or Chelsea, by contrast, I don't think that finishing fourth is such an achievement. With their finances, they should be challenging for the title. That's the difference: fourth is a fantastic achievement for a club like Everton, but a disappointment for some others.

Everton didn't just finish fourth in 2004–05, but have gone on to maintain a consistently high finish in the league pretty much ever since. In both 2007–08 and 2008–09, the club got more points than in 2004–05, but this was only enough for fifth. That consistency has been down to David, to the support he had from the chairman, and the players they brought in. During his time at the club, he developed a squad that was his, and was always looking to improve it with the right type of characters, and the right sort of players. Everton might not have the finances of some of our bigger rivals, but we make up for that in the thoroughness of our research. When we are scouting someone, we'll have him watched thirty, forty, fifty times. It is that in-depth, in order to make sure that we spend our money as wisely as we can.

David was clearly ambitious when he joined the club, but did he think he would be in a position to turn the club into a consistent top six team? Realistically, I would say no, though he would probably say different! Any team can have a fluke season – that happens both ways round. But if you are finishing in around the same position year after year, then that shows where you are as a club. Despite having comparatively limited resources, that is what David has achieved. Although there may be no trophy to show for it, anyone who knows football knows what a big deal that is. It was no surprise to me, then, when he was chosen to succeed Sir Alex Ferguson at Manchester United.

# 14

---

# Black Cats and More Toffees

At the end of the season that Everton qualified for the Champions League, my contract was up. Because of the push for fourth place, David didn't want to talk about it until the season was over. My agent, Paul Stretford, tried a couple of times to discuss it, but the club were firm that there would be no talks until after the season was finished. Which was fine – getting into the Champions League was the priority, and I was happy to wait.

The end of the season came, and the club offered me another contract. The money was good, that was never an issue. However, the contract was only for twelve months. It was club policy, I was told, that no player over thirty was offered more than a year's contract. I said immediately to both the club and my agent that I wouldn't be signing it. I felt that after the season I'd had, playing my part in getting the club into the Champions League, I warranted a two-year deal. The level of wages they were offering was never even discussed: I wanted to play for Everton. I would have stayed at Celtic if money was my priority, as they were paying good wages at the time.

David spoke to me, and told me that he wanted me to sign the contract.

'I'm not signing, Gaffer,' I told him, 'not unless I get another two years. I feel as if I deserve that.'

'I know,' David said, 'but it's club policy. We only offer one-year deals to players over thirty.'

'That's fine,' I replied. 'But if that is the policy, then I won't be signing.'

David continued to press me to sign, and told me to go away and think about it. But I was adamant: my decision would be the same whether it was May or when the contract ran out at the end of June. The club continued to ring and ask for an answer, but my position didn't change. I felt hurt, I've got to be honest. After such a really good season, I didn't want things to turn sour or negative. Maybe other players in my position would have signed the contract on the table, but I believed I deserved longer and stuck to my guns.

It was while this was going on that I was informed that the club were considering including a clause in the new contract regarding my previous battles with cancer: as I understood it, should I have a relapse and be diagnosed with cancer again, then they were legally entitled to terminate the contract. When I found out about that, I was very upset and disappointed. I'd probably played as many games as anyone had that season, and there was talk of some sort of cancer clause being put in for the following season.

I felt degraded. I thought to myself, just because I have had cancer, does that now mean I have to have a stigma attached to me for the rest of my life? It had been hard enough to go through those experiences: now it seemed as though people wanted to label me as different, for what I had been through. It just didn't make sense, and I still don't quite understand the reasons behind it. There hadn't been any such clause in my previous contract with the club. What's more I had a letter from my specialist to say that I was all clear.

I spoke to the Gaffer and to Keith Wyness, who was chief executive at the time, and told them what I thought. I think, looking back, that if the situation arose again, then everyone involved would probably have acted differently. I think that's true of the club, and it's also true of myself. I'm not exempting myself from how everything unfolded. Certainly, when I later returned to Everton, there was no clause regarding cancer in any of the subsequent contracts.

Having turned the contract down, I sat down with my agent to look at the other offers on the table. There were a couple of deals, but nothing immediately outstanding. That was to be expected: I was in my thirties, even if just having had one of the best seasons of my career. Going to Wolves was one possibility; Leeds United was another. Then Sunderland, who had been newly promoted under Mick McCarthy, made an offer. The money on the table was the same as what I had been offered at Everton and was for two years. I liked Mick, too, and so agreed to sign.

Right from the start, I found it difficult to settle at Sunderland. The family stayed in Liverpool, and I rented a big house on the Wynyard Estate, County Durham. I should have got myself a small apartment, but I wanted somewhere for the family to come up and stay at the weekend. During the week, I was rattling about on my own, and having to cook and look after myself. I didn't enjoy it.

I should say that I always thought there was a lot going for Sunderland. The people were great, very passionate about their team. The staff at the club and the training ground were fantastic. Mick, too, was someone I had a lot of time for. He was your classic straight-talking Yorkshireman: he pulled no punches and let everyone know exactly where they stood. The players gave their all for him, but it quickly became apparent that it wasn't going to be enough. They were young lads and some of them weren't ready for the Premier League, physically or mentally. There were a few of them who still liked to go out on the drink during the week. As a manager, that's difficult to control: if the players go out on a Tuesday, have Wednesday off and aren't back in until Thursday, then unless something gets in the papers, you don't know what's been going on. Certainly, Newcastle is a good night out, and some of those players made the most of it.

Quite early on, Mick pulled me into his office and said, 'This is going to be a really tough season, Alan.' Within a couple of months, he said that the signs weren't good that they were going to stay up. He told me that if I could find a club in the January transfer window, then they would let me go; if they were going down, they couldn't afford to keep me on the wages they were paying me.

Right at the end of December, Everton came to the Stadium of Light for a league match. I had a box at the time, and Mandy and the kids, and my best friend and his kids all came to watch the match. The box was towards the left-hand side of the dugout as you came out, right in the Sunderland end. I was on the bench that day, and it wasn't a great game. It was goalless until injury time, when Tim Cahill popped up to head home the winner. As soon as he scored, Mandy, my mate, his wife and all the kids jumped up and started celebrating. The next thing I knew, the media had put two and two together to make five, and the press was full of stories that *I* was the one who had been celebrating. It was just totally, totally wrong. You know what? If I had celebrated, hand on heart I would say so. I've got nothing to hide. But the truth didn't seem to matter: the story stuck. Whenever I went back to Sunderland later on in my career, I always got booed as a result, which was a shame.

While all of this was going on, Everton had had a terrible start to the season. Beset by injuries, they had even slid into the relegation places during the autumn. I was still in touch with various people at the club, and spoke to Jimmy Lumsden, the first-team coach, on a few occasions.

'What is it like?' he asked about Sunderland. 'Are you enjoying it?'

'Not really,' I said.

Then in one of the phone calls, he asked, 'would you consider coming back?'

Immediately, I said, 'I would love to.'

'Okay, Alan,' Jimmy replied. 'Leave it with me.'

Come the January transfer window, a meeting was set with David – it was at a hotel called the Tickled Trout, just off the M6 in Preston. It was great to see him, and straightaway he said, 'Everything that went on in the summer, can we a draw a line under it? If we can, then I'd love to bring you back.'

I agreed. 'I just want to play,' I said.

There was a contract on the table until the end of the season, with an agreement to look at the situation again after that. We also reached an agreement over a line to take about what had happened in the summer: if anyone asked, we'd simply say we had moved on. I was delighted to be returning. I had never wanted to leave in the first place.

My first game back came quicker than I was expecting. We were at home to Arsenal and David put me on the bench. After about half an hour, Matteo Ferrari, who had been playing at the back, had to come off with an injury. I was on, and was pleased to get a good response from the fans to my return. They knew I hadn't wanted to go and that circumstances had led to my leaving. I slotted back in alongside David Weir, and it was almost as if I had never been away. It was more as if I'd been out with an injury for four months, rather than playing for another team. The game was something of a baptism of fire – Arsenal had Thierry Henry up front, with Cesc Fabregas and Robert Pires in support – but we held out, and with James Beattie nicking a winner, we bagged the three points. Pretty soon, the threat of relegation was lifted and we ended up finishing the season in a respectable eleventh place.

In my second stint at Everton, the competition to play at the back was fierce: there was myself and David Weir, Joseph Yobo, and now also Joleon Lescott. Right at the end, there was Phil Jagielka too. They were all top, top players, which made getting a regular place in the starting XI a challenge.

One of David Moyes' goals was to bring down the age of the team. We were an ageing squad, to an extent, and the purchase of someone like Joleon was an attempt to rectify that. I wasn't stupid: David Weir and I were both well into our thirties and weren't going to be going on forever. The manager had to look ahead, buy and bed in some young blood to the team. It was a bit like when I was starting out my career at Bolton, except rather than being the young player, I was now the established one, offering experience and advice. And just like at Bolton, as friendly as we were to the new recruits, the older players were determined to cling onto their places.

Both David and I were in good form, and made it difficult for the Gaffer to leave either of us out, particularly as we worked so well as a unit. Joseph Yobo was a great player, very quick and brought something different to what we could do at the back, but he was also more of an individual and would only really worry about his own area on the pitch. There was quite often this 'three into two doesn't go' dilemma for the manager, and into this came Joleon. He'd been in fantastic form for Wolves and the club were delighted to sign him for £5 million. Joleon had been linked with a number of Premier League teams, but for some reason no one had tried to sign him: I don't know if there was a certain part of his game people weren't sure about, or whether it was a medical thing. Joleon had knee problems, and has to be careful how he manages them, so maybe that was it.

It quickly turned out to be the other teams' loss and Everton's gain. Joleon was a great lad to have around and settled in really well. He was quite quiet to begin with, off the pitch at least: he was happy to shout on the pitch. He was still maturing as a foot-baller, and playing alongside older players like David, Joseph and myself helped his game develop. With competition for the central defensive places being fierce, the Gaffer started playing Joleon at left-back to accommodate him: Joleon was a good enough player that he could adapt his game to play there, and with him on the flank, the back of the team had both balance and a strong look to it.

Phil Jagielka also came in. Like myself, and also Leighton Baines, he had been an Everton boy who was let go and had made it elsewhere. Jags had been playing for Sheffield United and was very much their star player. Sometimes it can be difficult to come from a club where you're the main man to another where you're just one of the squad, but Jags handled himself really well. Like Joleon, he didn't get to play in central defence immediately: the manager had him at right-back, and also in midfield: wherever we were short.

It was clear, though, that the centre of defence was where Joleon and Jags' future lay. I couldn't begrudge them that: they are both top quality players and deservedly went on to become England internationals. But at the same time, there were consequences for me. After the season when I returned, I signed another year long contract, and the club had a great season and finished sixth. I signed again for another year, and in the first half of the season, the team continued this decent form.

I was delighted for the team, though disappointed not to be getting as much game time as I'd have liked. I knew I wasn't going to be playing every week, but even so, I wanted to play as much as possible. I discussed it with the Gaffer, and he told me that I needed to play for as long as I could.

'Once you hang your boots up,' David said, 'that's it. So the longer you can play on for, the better.'

I hadn't been looking to go, but in the January transfer window, an offer came in from Derby County. I chatted to David about what to do, and he was great about it.

'It is entirely up to you,' he said. 'If you want to stay here, you are more than welcome. But obviously, this is a chance for you to play as well.'

The offer from Derby was a difficult one to turn down: it was an eighteen-month contract, twenty grand a week, with no relegation clause in it. Derby at the time had just been promoted to the Premier League, and were struggling to stay up. It was good money, and manager Paul Jewell wanted to bring me in as his captain to try and steady the ship. I discussed it with David, and his advice was clear: I'd be stupid not to take it. It meant I would be playing regularly, and the contract would probably take me to the end of my career. So we shook hands on it, and I went off and signed.

My last club, Derby County, was another with both a bit of history to it and a loyal, passionate fanbase: thirty-odd thousand fans a week, you can't complain about that. The whole set-up was geared for the Premier League. It was just a shame that the results weren't happening on the pitch. Once again, as with both Bolton and Sunderland, there was not quite enough quality in the squad.

Paul Jewell had just taken over as manager from Billy Davies, who'd been sacked after a poor start to the season, and really wanted to do well. He'd already managed clubs like Wigan and Bradford but the Derby job was a big one, with potential for the person who got it right. I liked Paul a lot: he was a Scouser, and his passion for the job was there for all to see. He was the sort of guy who never hid what he was feeling, and it was clear to everyone that he felt frustrated and under pressure to get results. That came from a good place – he wanted it to work so badly – but the upshot was that the players often got it in the neck. When Paul came out for training, the team would all be looking over, to gauge what sort of mood he was in.

Paul was great with me, but there were one or two in the squad who were a bit less sure about him. When players don't like a manager, it's usually because they're not being picked. Simple as that. Robbie Savage was one of those: he was great when he was in the team, but a nuisance when he wasn't. There was plenty of friction between him and Paul when he wasn't selected. Robbie thought he should be in the team and was better than the players who had been chosen instead. He wasn't shy in telling Paul that in front of the other players.

I really liked Robbie and got on well with him. He could have taken the hump with me because he had been captain and had to hand his armband over, but we always got on. We were the experienced players, both getting towards the end of our careers, and both wanting to play games. I didn't disagree with Robbie's assessment of whether or not he should have been in the team, but I did think there was a time and a place for such comments. For me, Robbie didn't always choose the right moment to vent his feelings.

Robbie was the sort of player who needed an arm round the shoulder. He was quite insecure, and as much as he would tell everyone how good he was, needed to be told that as well. But having been so openly critical of the manager, he wasn't going to get that love back from him. Robbie was quite vocal in his negative comments by the end, and that just exacerbated the situation.

There was an element too, here, of a player coming to terms with the end of his career. Any footballer in their final years is not going to be the player that they once were. That can be hard to take, and some players cope with it better than others. Some, and I think Robbie was one, struggle to accept it. More than anything, it's that lack of speed that gets you – you're not as fast as you once were, and hard as you might try, you don't get to the second balls in the same way. Robbie's game was never one about getting the ball and passing it; his was all about closing people down and basically being a pain in the arse for the opposition. To pull it off, that's high energy stuff. Robbie was desperate to convince us he could still do it. On the training ground, he'd be tackling and getting in people's faces, all the while shouting little comments across to Paul. 'See? Who says I can't keep doing this?'

I could feel I was getting on as well. Throughout my entire time at Derby, I don't think I was ever one hundred per cent fit. I had a knee injury – a ball of fluid, a sort of cyst – that needed dealing with. I had it cleared out, which helped for a while, but then the problem returned. It was painful to play through. The knee injury stopped me from jumping and competing in the air, and hindered me from turning quickly. I was very conscious of it when I was playing – once you're thinking like that, then that detracts from your focus on the game.

I didn't have any cortisone injections, or anything like that: just treatment, ice and scans. I could have rested it for six to eight weeks to try and clear it up, but I felt uncomfortable doing that. By this point, we were well into training for the new season. Derby had been relegated down to the Championship, and the manager had a fight on his hands to take the team back up. The last thing I wanted was to be a hindrance to that.

I went to see Paul and said to him, 'I don't know whether I'm going to be fit for you.'

'Why don't you try giving the knee a rest?' Paul suggested. 'See how it feels after a few weeks.'

'I would do,' I said, 'but what I'm trying to say is that I could rest for six to eight weeks, and then in eight weeks' time when you're expecting me to play, I might be saying it's still not ready and I need another couple of months. You can't constantly have a situation where you're unsure whether you'll be back next week or not.'

I wanted to be fair to Paul. He'd been good with me and I wanted to give him the best possible chance of succeeding at the club. It would have been the easiest thing in the world to sit out the end of my contract, and just take the money. But it wouldn't have been right. I knew that if I went, then he'd have the opportunity to bring someone else in instead.

I had this discussion with Paul, and went on to see the club chairman, Adam Pearson. Adam was a really good guy, my sort of bloke, and I always enjoyed working with him. I explained the situation to him, told him that it wasn't happening, and asked if there was any way we could sort things out. No problem, Adam said. We reached an agreement on the rest of my contract and settled everything extremely amicably.

I think for a lot of players when they retire, it can feel as though their world has caved in. For me, from what I had been through with the cancer, it didn't seem a big deal. There was going to be a part of me that missed the football, and playing on a Saturday

afternoon and midweek, but deciding to quit wasn't as big a decision as for some players. In fact, my mind had been made up
about it pretty quickly. I'd had a discussion about it with Mandy,
and with a few a friends in football, but I was very clear about it
from the start. I suspect it is a decision that is easier to take today
than it was twenty or thirty years ago, because football is a well-
paid profession these days, and the financial impact of retiring is
not what it once was. But even so, there are plenty of examples of
footballers who finish their careers and go on the drink or off the
rails – they struggle without the routine of training and end up
piling on the pounds. I wasn't sure what I was going to do, but I
was determined to avoid that.

A couple of weeks later, I had to drop in at Everton to pick up a
signed shirt for someone. While I was there, I bumped into David
Moyes, who asked how I was. He knew just how much playing on
had meant to me. I was okay about it, I told him. I might go away on
holiday and take a little time to reflect, but basically I was all right.

'What are your plans?' David asked.

Beyond the holiday, I hadn't really thought. David asked how
long I was staying for, and asked if I'd mind hanging around for
a couple of hours. He had a press conference to do, but would like
to have a chat with me. I said, sure, I'll wait, and went round to
say hello to various players and staff. Then the press conference
finished and David called me into his office.

'What do you want to do?' David asked again. 'Have you
thought about staying in football?'

What *were* my plans? I knew that one day I wanted to be a
manager, but quite how I'd go down that route I hadn't really
thought through at that point.

David asked about my coaching badges and I told him where I
was at: I'd done my 'B' badge, and was doing my 'A' and 'Pro' licence.

'If you want,' David offered, 'you can come here and coach. I'll make a role available.'

When David said this, I was a little taken aback. It was an amazing offer, but was still only a week after I'd retired. David told me to go away and think about it. I saw him on the Friday, and he suggested I gave him a call back on the Monday. I went away and had a chat with Andrew 'Taff' Holden, the reserve-team manager. I told Taff what David had offered, and he was very welcoming.

'Come in and work alongside me,' he said. 'I'll help you and show you the ropes.'

On the Monday, I rang David back and told him that I'd like to give it a go.

'Great,' David said. 'I'll see you tomorrow.'

And that was it. Within a fortnight of retiring from playing, I was back in, and beginning my career as a coach.

Going into coaching had always been something I'd been interested in doing, and towards the end of my playing career had taken my 'B' licence. The course to get the licence took place over seven days, with a further five days a little later on. I took the course in Stockport, and although I passed it, didn't particularly enjoy the experience. The course wasn't great, and one of the coaches taking it was a little awkward towards the ex-players doing it: as well as myself, there was also the likes of Jason Wilcox and Dean Richards, who sadly is no longer with us. I don't know whether the coach, who had also been a player, felt the game owed him something. But it wasn't a good atmosphere, and some of the players, including Jason, left the course.

When you do a course like that as a player, you do feel quite vulnerable. This was the first time most of us had done any form of coaching, and it was 'in at the deep end' stuff. On top of this, you had to put sessions on in front of your fellow professionals, and that was quite a daunting task. It was quite weird giving advice to seasoned pros – you might be taking a session on striker movement and find yourself telling a prolific goalscorer that he should be doing something a bit different. Everyone was very good humoured about it, though, as they knew they'd have to run a similar session themselves. 'Are you sure about that, Alan?' they'd say with a smile and a wink.

There was about eighteen or so of us in the group. There were footballers who were still playing, some who'd retired, and also amateur players and those who worked for local clubs and in the community. It was an interesting mix. Although I was slightly uncertain about the course, I really enjoyed the coaching itself. I learned a lot: as a player, you can be quite oblivious and ignorant to the preparation that has gone on before a session. You turn up, see it all set-up and think, oh, we're doing that today. Find your-self on the other side, and you realise how much thought it actu-ally involved. A particular session might have been chosen because of the team's opposition the following week. To decide what training might be useful involves watching and analysing how the other team play. That's quite a lot of work and needs doing in advance: you can't just turn up to the training ground on the day and wing it.

At the 'B' licence level, the game is broken up into what are called functions and phases of play. Functions would be things like passing, crossing and finishing; phases of play could be areas like attacking, counterattacking, midfield runs or wide play. You think of the game in terms of these sorts of topic and try to devise training sessions that reflected them. At the 'A' licence level, you look at these in more depth: you watch a game and analyse it; you are shown how to create a pre-season programme, structuring a timetable of high intensity, low intensity and rest sessions. You'd look again at phases of play in more detail and work on team shape. So for example, you might be working on the full-backs overlapping: you'd begin with a session of 11 vs 8, in order to give the full-backs space to practise. Then you'd build this up to an 11 vs 11 game, when hopefully the overlapping would be working, and the team was keeping its shape.

The 'A' licence is a much longer course. It takes place over twelve months, with an initial session of nine days, followed by two to three-day sessions during the year, and another week to finish at the end. I took mine at Largs in Scotland, where I also went on to take my 'Pro' Licence. It was David Moyes who suggested I went up there to do it, after the disappointment of the 'B' licence course in England. It was a great recommendation: Largs is *the* place to learn to coach and the course boasts some amazing alumni: David did the course there, as did Jose Mourinho and Andre Villas-Boas. It's got that high a reputation.

Having done my 'A' licence, I went on to study for my 'Pro' Licence. This takes about twenty months to complete and was less focused on the coaching side and more to do with the practicalities of management. I did sessions on transfers, where you would practise negotiating with agents. We looked at job interviews, where they got board members of St Mirren to come in and give you the sort of grilling you'd get.

A section of the course was about scouting and match analysis. The whole course – about twenty-four of us – went over to the Under-21 Championships, which that year was being held in Denmark. There would be different topics every day – weaknesses, opposition strength, style of play – and each evening you'd be put into groups and have to put together a PowerPoint presentation to show your thoughts. Some of the guys on the course had never so much as switched a computer on, so that was a challenge. We were up until three or four in the morning getting the presentations right.

Because of its reputation, Largs is great at getting managers coming to speak at the course. Sir Alex Ferguson, Andre Villas-Boas, Marcello Lippi and Lars Lagerback were just some of the names who came to speak to us. The sessions were all off the record, and were on the understanding that what was said would stay in the room. So I can't reveal anything about what I was told! But the result was that you had these top managers being fantastically frank about their careers and their players. It was eye-opening stuff.

The course was quite intense at the time, but the 'Pro' Licence has been invaluable: some of the stuff you were taught you might have had a fair idea of already, but plenty of it wouldn't have crossed my mind otherwise. And it has been useful and practical – I've used what I learned a lot in my coaching. It's a mandatory qualification, now, if you want to manage in the Premier League, but even if it wasn't it would have been well worth doing.

I have really enjoyed my coaching, right from the beginning. It is like I have gone back full circle, and am a little kid starting something new. From the start, Everton were brilliant with me: Taff, in particular, I couldn't thank enough. He really let me find my own feet. He'd let me take a bit of the training session, watch over me, and tell me what I was doing right or wrong afterwards. After a while, when I'd learned the basics, he'd say, 'Why don't you take the session today?' and just observe.

I'd try and tap into my experience and ability as a footballer, and attempt to bring those skills and knowledge across to the management side. But there is still plenty to learn: even though I've been a defender, say, there is still stuff I can learn about how to coach defending. I quickly realised that it wasn't just what you know, but how you get this information across to your players. I remembered as a player that the coach would try and tell you something, and you'd just nod as though you knew what he was saying, even though you didn't.

Now I was the coach, I had to get past this. Every player, you realise, is different. You have some bright ones, intelligent in a football sense, who can take instructions on board on the first go. You have some thick players too, so that requires a different way of getting the message across. You have players, too, who struggle with concentration – you can see as you're instructing them that they're starting to switch off. So there's always a lot of tailoring going on: there's no point running a really technical and tactical session if the players don't understand it.

As the 2012–13 season came to its close, I had been coaching the reserves, or the Under-21s as the league is called these days, for four years. We'd had a good season, and were preparing to play Tottenham in the semi-final of the competition when everything at Everton was turned on its head. Rumours started circulating that Sir Alex Ferguson was about to retire as Manchester United manager. Once it was officially announced, the talk immediately turned to who his successor might be: David Moyes was quickly touted as a possible candidate.

I was at the club when I saw Sir Alex's retirement flashed up as being official on Sky Sports News. I went into the coaches' room, where I saw David, and told him what I'd seen on the TV.

'Yeah, I know,' he said. 'I knew about that the other day. Listen, I can't say much, but there is something going on. But I need to speak to the chairman first before I say anything.'

David told me later that when he had been invited to see Sir Alex, he'd thought it had been to discuss the possibility of Leighton Baines or Marouane Fellaini moving to Old Trafford. But it was David moving there that Sir Alex had wanted to talk about. If you want it, the job's yours, he was told.

It goes without saying that everyone at Everton was hugely disappointed to see David go. But it was a fantastic opportunity for him, and one that his talents as a manager deserved. I'd been at Everton for pretty much his whole tenure at the club, first as a player and then as a coach. Seeing him work at first hand, there's no doubt in my mind that he has long been one of the top two or three managers in the country. As a young coach, I've learned so much from David over the years, and will always remain grateful for the chances he has given me, both on and off the pitch.

Once the news was out, the end of the season was a bit of a strange one at Everton. It turned into a bit of a media circus, with photographers hanging about outside the training ground and every journalist under the sun wanting a seat at the press conference. On the training ground, there was something of a surreal atmosphere: David wanted the team to put in a good performance over the last couple of matches, not just for him, but for them, too, for all the hard work they'd put in over the season. It was business as usual, and yet it wasn't at the same time.

The final match at Goodison was a memorable occasion. There were a few nerves around beforehand, and no one was quite sure what the reception was going to be: there were a few fans who were saying things like, well if he is going, why is he still here? In the end, though, the worries were unfounded: the fans gave David the send-off he deserved. He got an amazing response from the supporters, and one that befitted both him and the club. It was one of those occasions that make you proud to be an Evertonian.

The next question on everyone's lips was who would replace him as manager. When I first learned that David was leaving, it didn't initially cross my mind to apply for the job. But the more I thought about it, the more I wanted to put my name forwards: I knew the club and set-up inside out, and felt ready to step up after my time with the Under-21s. As it happened, I was down in London with the Under-21s for the Tottenham match, which is where the chairman has his offices. So I took the opportunity of asking if we could meet up to discuss it.

The chairman was great. We had an informal chat about the role, and had a really good discussion about Everton, about me, and about the club going forwards. The only people I told about the meeting were Mandy and my best mate, yet as the days went on, I saw my name starting to rise up the betting odds. I started getting besieged with messages and calls from people, guys claiming they knew someone who knew someone, and they'd heard I'd got the job. It was all rumour, and without foundation, and I stopped answering the calls in the end.

Before he offered the job to Roberto Martinez, the chairman rang to tell me that he had decided not to go internal with the appointment. He didn't have to do that, and I appreciated his doing so. He didn't tell me it was going to be Roberto, though – if he had, I'd have been down the bookies myself! For all Roberto's achievements of winning the FA Cup, it was probably Wigan's defeat of Everton in the quarter-final that made the chairman sit up and take notice of him: it wasn't a great day for Everton, but quite a calling card for Roberto.

I was disappointed not to get the job, of course. I do believe that management is something I'd be good at, and if the right opportunity comes along, I'll be ready to have a crack at it. But at the same time, there's no doubt that Roberto is a great appointment, both for the club and also in my ongoing development as a young coach. The way I see it is that here's another fantastic manager that I can learn from. I'm really looking forward to working with Roberto, and helping him to build on David's legacy and take Everton forwards. Right now, there's nowhere else I'd rather be.

Back in the summer, the hardback edition of this book went to print soon after Roberto took over at Everton and David Moyes departed for Manchester United. Six months down the line, it has been fascinating to see how Goodison has responded to new management.

At Everton, it was certainly a case of a fresh start at Finch Farm. Not only did David leave for Old Trafford, but so too did a whole number of support staff, from the goalkeeping coach to the scouting team. That's how management works these days: it's not just about the man in charge, but that core team of individuals who help out in so many different ways. Roberto has been no different, bringing with him the likes of Graeme Jones, Dennis Lawrence and Richard Evans as part of his coaching staff.

No disrespect to Wigan, but moving to Everton from there was a shift up in terms of scale for Roberto, and in terms in the number of staff (no different, in all honesty, for David going to Manchester United). We're a big club and that can take a little bit of time to adjust to. Equally, Everton had to adjust to a new man in charge after such a long spell under the previous gaffer. What we have discovered is a guy who brings a more laidback attitude to the job compared to David's intensity, but one whose hard work and attention to detail are phenomenal. Roberto is very thorough in his research and his analysis: he is incredibly meticulous and, right from the word go, I've been hugely impressed by his knowledge and understanding of the game.

I've also been impressed by the amount of freedom he has given me to coach the Under-21s. Sometimes, a new manager asks for the sides down the age groups to play in a similar style, so if a player is called up to the next level, they can quickly slot in to the same system. Roberto, by contrast, has a more open-minded approach. His main request has been for the players to be flexible, to be able to adapt to play in different formations. The other main change has been to allow me to create my own team, in an echo of the first team set-up – rather than sharing staff across the club as we used to, now the Under-21s have our own physio, sports scientist and so on. I've also got David Unsworth in as assistant manager and it's been great to be back working with him again.

Roberto's approach has been rewarded with a fantastic first few months as manager of Everton on the pitch. The new players he has brought in – the likes of James McCarthy, Gareth Barry, Romelu Lukaku and Gerard Deulofeu – have adjusted well and brought both a stability and vibrancy to the team's play. Although Lukaku has been getting the headlines, as strikers always do, for me Gareth Barry has been the best signing of the lot. He's a top pro, a great trainer and has a calmness and quiet authority to him that is hard not to admire. He's fantastic to have around.

And then there's Ross Barkley. Ross has become a permanent fixture in the team this season and, as someone who has worked with him over the last two or three years and watched him develop, I couldn't be more delighted for him. Particularly as that progression has been hampered by a number of nasty injuries – in the space of 18 months, Ross had a double leg fracture, a double hernia and a broken metatarsal. Faced with all that, a player can start to question things, whether or not it is meant to be. Ross, to his absolute credit, wasn't put off by that at all. He got knocked down and got up again, as the song goes. And each time he has come back stronger. He's a diamond lad, and a real star in the making.

People are always asking me who Ross reminds me of: is he the new Gazza, the new Gerrard, the new Wayne? I think he's got to be given time to find his own identity, rather than seeing him in terms of those who have come before him. Yes, there are bits of all kinds of great players in his play: there's something of the way he runs off people that reminds me of Gazza, he has the sense of belonging on a football pitch the way Steven Gerrard does. But with Ross the package is different and he's going to develop still further before he's the finished product.

The breakthrough of Ross is a good riposte to those who think that England can't produce great young players in the way that other countries can. Ross has the capacity to do great things and in Roberto he's got the perfect person to nurture that talent. It's exciting for Everton and for the national side as well. Watching him turn out at Goodison, it reminds me why I got into coaching in the first place – one of those moments when the future of English football looks bright after all.

# Epilogue

It probably started for my dad when he fell off his bike. I don't quite know why he came off. He hadn't been hit by anyone, wasn't feeling dizzy or anything like that. But whether he was turning a corner, hit a stone or whatever, he lost his balance and hit the ground. He wasn't particularly hurt by it, but it seemed to be quite a significant moment: after that, he went on a downward spiral that he never quite seemed to recover from. The fall just seemed to knock the stuffing out of him.

My dad was a really proud man. He was your old fashioned sort of guy who did not want to go to the doctors if he could avoid it at all. He wouldn't tell anyone if he was unwell: he would just get on with it until it went away. The only time he'd see the GP was as a last resort, or if he needed something specifically, like blood pressure tablets. He was a fit and healthy man; he'd smoked when he was younger, but gave them up after he'd had a heart attack. He stopped smoking instantly.

After the bicycle fall, my dad had started to look a little frail. He was complaining, which wasn't like him at all, that things were not right. He was complaining of a dry throat the whole time. We took him in to see the doctor and the hospital to have tests done: I was fairly well versed by this point as to what they would do. I remember being with my older sister Susan at the hospital, as the doctor came back with the results. I asked him to tell us the full extent of the situation.

The doctor was straight with us. It was cancer, and my father had it all over his body: his stomach, his bowel, his chest, he was riddled with it. I asked how long he had, and the doctor said six months, if that. We were both devastated. Susan was really upset, and I remember putting my arms around her and giving her a hug. I was the youngest in the family, but I knew I had to be the strong one. Because I'd been through it, I knew what to do and how to respond to it.

It was so soon since I'd recovered myself from cancer. This happened right at the start of my first season with Everton: I'd barely come down from Scotland and it was a lot to take in. When I look back now, I am glad for my dad's sake that it happened so quickly. He knew he wasn't well, my dad. He wasn't soft. He would have been fighting it, even before he was diagnosed. When he went to the hospital, it was when he probably couldn't bear it any longer. It was good, looking back, that he didn't have to suffer for long.

Dad was of the generation who found it difficult to talk about what he was feeling. As I say, he was a proud man. On one occasion, I remember him being back at the house and I was there with my mate John. John and my dad were together in the back room watching telly, and I was out of the room doing something else. Dad had lost a lot of weight by this point: it was painful to see.

Once I was out of the room, he turned to John and said to him, 'I'm taking it. I want to take all the cancer from Alan. I'm going to take it all with me so that he is all right.'

That was him all over. There's no way Dad could have said that to me directly; he would have broken down, trying to say that to me. I was in tears when John told me what he'd said. It was typical of my father – selfless to the last. He would do anything for his family. Anything.

When the end came, I had been away playing with Everton. I was on the way back from the match and got a call from Mandy. She rang to ask me if I'd spoken to Susan. Straightaway, I think I realised what had probably happened. I rang Susan, and she just told me to get to the hospital as quickly as I could.

I turned the car round and put my foot down. I've probably never driven so fast, or probably as recklessly. I just wanted to get there. I reached the hospital and raced into reception, where Susan was waiting. As soon as I saw her, I knew.

'He's passed away, hasn't he?' I asked.

Susan just nodded.

I went upstairs: I wanted to see him. There was a private room where my family all were: my mum, my sisters, my brothers-in-law. I gave my mum a hug, and said that I wanted to see my dad. The others made a move to come to the ward with me, but I stopped them. I wanted a couple of minutes by myself. I went up to the ward where he was, and the curtains were all drawn around the bed. I pulled them back, and then pulled back the blankets on the bed so I could see him. It was probably the wrong thing to do, to be honest. He had deteriorated so fast and had lost so much weight, it didn't look like him at all. That's not my dad, I thought to myself. That was what the cancer had done to him. It was devastating. It was worse than when I'd been told I had cancer. That news didn't affect me the way that losing my dad did.

*   *   *

I may have overcome cancer myself, but despite having been all clear ever since, I've never been too far away from the pain it can cause. In 2006, Tommy Burns, who'd taken me to Celtic when he was manager, started receiving treatment for skin cancer. In 2008, he too sadly died from the disease: he was only fifty-one. I went up to Scotland for the funeral and it was an extraordinary occasion. It hit home just how much of a legend Tommy was in Scotland, not just among the Celtic fans, but way beyond that.

The streets were lined with people for his funeral. Space in the church was so oversubscribed that the players who wanted to attend had to tell the club that they were coming, because so many of us wanted to. The then manager Gordon Strachan and the entire current first-team squad were there: Martin O'Neill, Roy Keane, David Moyes and Walter Smith were just some of the many others; Tommy's former team-mates Pat Bonner, Danny McGrain, Peter Grant and George McCluskey brought the coffin in. Alex Salmond, the Scottish First Minister was there too, emphasising just what a major occasion it was.

After the service, we went to the crematorium and then back to Celtic Park. Mandy and I wanted to see Tommy's wife, Rosemary and the kids; she had been so kind to us when we first moved up and had helped us to settle. They are a lovely family, and I would not have expected anything different because of the man. TB, as we used to call him, was a top bloke and a real gentleman: there's not many people you can say that about as a manager. He was charismatic, had this infectious personality, and that's how I'll always remember him. It was a privilege to know him.

Tommy's death from cancer wasn't the only one to touch me in recent years: a young member of my family also tragically died of leukaemia. It was desperately sad, and all happened so quickly. She had been complaining of cold-like symptoms, so her mother took her to see her doctor on the Wednesday. The doctor sent her to hospital and by that evening she had a couple of blood tests and been diagnosed with the disease, a really aggressive form of it. The doctors gave her an intensive course of chemotherapy to try to overcome it. The whole family were there in the hospital every day, hoping she would be okay. But on the Sunday she died.

To lose someone like that, it is indescribable. Sometimes it feels as though cancer had taken a grip on my family. That was three generations: my father, me, and now her. Every corner we turned, it seemed to take a loved one. Cancer is one of those illnesses where you end up asking yourself more questions than you get answers. It would be very easy for me to look at everything that has gone on and say, why me? Why my dad? Why her? They say that God moves in mysterious ways; when it comes to cancer, it can seem an extremely mysterious way indeed.

I am just so fortunate that I am here to be able to tell my story. After everything I have been through, I would be happy if I was to make it to fifty, to sixty, seventy, whatever. I hope and pray that I can have a full parenthood with my children, and that they never end up in the same situation that I was in, or my dad. I would not wish that on anyone.

What keeps me going is the fact that I have never felt sorry for myself: not when I was given the original diagnosis, not since. I felt sorry for my dad. I certainly felt sorry for my family. But as far as I am concerned, I don't dwell. I look forward. I don't look back. And that's the way I'll always be.

One of the things I am proudest of in my life is that Dad got to see me play for Everton. To see me walking out at Goodison to make my debut was the biggest thing I could have done for him. It was something that I'd always dreamed of, but it was something that he'd dreamed of as well. For me to fulfil that, not just for me personally but for my dad too, was the best present I could ever have given him. After he'd gone, I'd play at Goodison, and would catch myself looking up to the stands.

It was as if there was an empty seat up there where my dad would have been sitting.

# Acknowledgements

This book would not have been possible without the support of family and friends. So heartfelt thanks to the following: my loving wife Mandy; my two special children, Heather and Sam, who have grown up so fast and made us very proud; my mum and my dad who made me what I am (Dad, I miss you so much); brother Ronnie and sisters Susan, Pam, Mandy who said I was always the spoilt one (ha ha); my great mates J Doolan, Boo, Ian and Mike McComb for being there when I needed them and for the laughs we've shared; all my team-mates who I have had the pleasure of knowing and playing with, the managers and their staff; and Professor Peter Clarke for all the help and reassurance he has provided since 2001 in our annual meetings at Clatterbridge Hospital.

I would also like to thank the following people for their help in putting this book together: Laura Doyle at Stellar and Zoe King at the Blair Partnership; Ian Marshall, Tom Whiting and everyone at Simon & Schuster; and Tom Bromley who has unearthed things about me that I would never of remembered or believed I did and made it very enjoyable to write.

# Index